PRIME TIME

A Doctor's Guide to Staying Younger Longer

JOHN E. EICHENLAUB, M.D.

PRENTICE HALL
Englewood Cliffs, New Jersey 07632

Prentice-Hall International (UK) Limited, *London*
Prentice-Hall of Australia Pty. Limited, *Sydney*
Prentice-Hall Canada, Inc., *Toronto*
Prentice-Hall Hispanoamericana, S.A., *Mexico*
Prentice-Hall of India Private Limited, *New Delhi*
Prentice-Hall of Japan, Inc., *Tokyo*
Simon & Schuster Asia Pte. Ltd., *Singapore*
Editora Prentice-Hall do Brasil, Ltda., *Rio de Janeiro*

© 1993 *by*

PRENTICE HALL

Englewood Cliffs, NJ

No book can replace the services of a trained physician. This book is not
intended to encourage treatment of illness, disease or other medical problems
by the layman. Any application of the recommendations set forth in the following
pages is at the reader's discretion and sole risk. If you are under a physician's
care for any condition, he or she can advise you about information described
in this book.

10 9 8 7 6 5 4 3 2 1

Library of Congress Cataloging-in-Publication Data

Eichenlaub, John E.
   Prime time : a doctor's guide to staying younger longer / by John E.
Eichenlaub, M.D.
     p. cm.
   Includes index.
   ISBN 0–13–435306–4 — ISBN 0-13-435298-X (pbk.)
   1. Aged—health and hygiene. I. Title.
RA777.6.E33   1993
613′.0438—dc20   92–30821
                                             CIP

ISBN 0-13-435298-X (PBK)

ISBN 0-13-435306-4

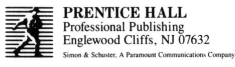

PRENTICE HALL
Professional Publishing
Englewood Cliffs, NJ 07632
Simon & Schuster, A Paramount Communications Company

Printed in the United States of America

Dedication

**To my wife Pat
whose delightful prime goes on and on.**

Acknowledgments

For years my wife Pat urged me to write this book, and I thank her for her ongoing encouragement. My editor, Deborah Kurtz, has a rare talent for helping an author do it better *his* way instead of imposing a style of her own, and made many valuable suggestions. Both by example and by discourse, David Torbett, Ph.D., deserves credit for many of the ideas in Chapter 23. Drs. Valerie Crandall Moore and Kim Spear read and made helpful comments with regard to the sections which involve their specialties.

Contents

What This Book Will Do for You

Think about age and how it will affect you.

Every year the numbers advance—you can't help that. But do you need to *feel* or *look* or *act* older? Can't you keep (or even improve) your capacities, widen your horizons instead of letting them shrink, and maintain your self-esteem?

You can keep old age at bay with the "divide and conquer" technique: fight off its harmful effects one at a time. If you *feel, look,* and *act* younger as the years go by, you'll have given the lie to the numbers, stayed younger longer, and effectively stretched your prime. That's what this book is all about.

Moreover, you don't need to become a slave to "doctor's orders," give up your favorite foods and activities, or devote endless hours to exercise to benefit from *Prime Time.* Along with practical, simple solutions to health and life-style problems, I've generally provided ways to choose minimal measures to suit your own needs. I don't just tell you how to keep your arteries pliable, for instance; I explain how you can tell which methods *you* need in view of your own background and habits. Likewise, I tell you how to work out *your own* osteoporosis proneness index and make just enough changes in your diet and activities to keep *your* bones sturdy.

What can a book help you do about advancing age?

First, it can help you ward off its erosion. The first twelve chapters tell you how to do that: how to keep your arteries supple and your bones sturdy, how to avoid or deal with hemorrhoids, hearing loss, gum disease, aging skin and nails, and sexual problems. In these chapters, I give concrete techniques for fighting off many of the ailments and conditions associated with "old age." These methods should help you build a sound foundation of physical and mental health on which to build an even better and more satisfying life-style as the years go by.

But holding your own isn't enough. The next four chapters tell you how to widen your horizons. They provide suggestions for adding more friends, more experiences, more energy, and more mind power to your life. They introduce simple techniques for meeting new people and making new friends, traveling more frequently and more comfortably, sharpening your memory, and getting a better night's sleep.

Even so, you can't ward off all the problems the passing years might bring. The final chapters of this book tell you how to handle those you're most likely to encounter. I've included home remedies for the types of headache, arthritis and rheumatism, back and neck pain, and breathing difficulties that commonly afflict people over age fifty. In particular I've stressed three subjects most books gloss over: how to heal injuries and recover your capacities afterward, how to adjust medications and habits to changing sensitivities, and how to cope with loss of dear ones or of crucial capacities and prerogatives.

While my emphasis is on things you can do for yourself, I've included some "early detection" aids, meant to get you to professional help when early care might be crucial. Two self-test charts help you to identify serious eye conditions, for example. Glancing at these every month will help you to find glaucoma or macular degeneration in its earliest stages. Prompt treatment of either condition often makes a huge difference to your future vision.

As a family doctor, I've always tried to know my limitations. If patients would benefit from something only a specialist could do, I've always told them so. The same applies here: you can do a lot for yourself with home measures, but it's still important to know when home measures aren't enough. I've tried to recommend a visit with your doctor whenever I believe that will give you further help.

All the solutions in *Prime Time* are "tried and true." With only occasional updating modifications, they're based on the experience of the hundreds of patients and friends I've treated or advised during the many years that I practiced medicine. I've shared their stories with you to give you an idea of how other people have dealt with some of the same issues and concerns you face.

In writing this book, I've tried to offer you the most effective available techniques for streching your prime. I hope the measures I've suggested work as well for you as they have for my patients and friends, as well as for me. I've used a great many of these methods myself, and I've stayed active into my seventies—and am still going strong! Just remember: you don't have to "get old" as the years pass. Take this book's lessons to heart, and you can stave off many elements of "old age." You can enjoy *Prime Time*'s comfort and vigor for many additional years.

CHAPTER

========= 1 =========

How to Keep Your Arteries Supple

Your number one priority for staying younger longer is to keep your arteries supple. This single step will help you avoid some of the most common problems of old age, from those of cold feet and poor memory to stroke and heart attack.

Accumulated cholesterol causes arteriosclerosis, or hardening of the arteries. But very little of that cholesterol comes directly from your foods. Your body forms almost all its cholesterol *inside* your body instead of taking it in from the *outside*. Eighty-five percent of the cholesterol in your system forms in the process of digesting the fats you eat, not from cholesterol-containing foods.

That's why you needn't spend very much of your willpower on limiting cholesterol. Just avoid real excess; then devote your main efforts to the other measures we'll discuss.

PRIME STRETCHER 1

*Pay attention to fats and oils rather than
cholesterol.*

Most health-conscious people focus on eliminating cholesterol and they neglect other, more important, factors in arteriosclerosis control.

STEP ONE: Limit cholesterol intake only moderately. Just keep it under 300 milligrams (mg.) per day. Unless you've had a heart attack or stroke or suffer from very high blood cholesterol readings,[1] all you need to do is keep your total cholesterol intake *under 300 mg. per day.* If you're a woman, chances are you're already within this limit; 300 mg. is the national average for women. The norm for men is 450 mg., but you shouldn't find it too difficult to cut your cholesterol intake by one-third. Remember that almost all the cholesterol in poultry is in the skin which you can discard, and that vegetables, grains, and fruits have no cholesterol at all.

Foods with 200 mg. Cholesterol

1 egg yolk	8 ounces lean veal
1 chocolate eclair	4 ounces steamed shrimp
2 ounces beef liver	5 ounces sardines in oil
6 ounces lean beef	1 chicken breast (with skin)
2 ounces pork liver	1/4 cup chicken liver
8 ounces lean pork	8 ounces turkey (with skin)

STEP TWO: Keep eggs on your menu. Egg whites are a great source of low-fat protein, so don't eliminate eggs from your diet. But two or more yolks will carry you over the recommended cholesterol limit, so limit yourself to one whole egg a day. You can make a tasty omelet or dish of scrambled eggs by using two egg whites for each whole egg. (If it bothers you to waste the yolks, feed them to your own or a neighbor's pet.)

Eat angel food cake and other baked goods that are made with egg whites and no yolk; they have almost no cholesterol.

---

[1] If you have any of these conditions, you probably have a diet that your doctor has prescribed especially for you. This may be more stringent than what I recommend for the usual reader.

You can keep your cholesterol intake in the appropriate range with very little effort. That leaves you with a lot of unused willpower to use where it really counts: on fats!

PRIME STRETCHER 2

Eat less saturated ("bad") fat or oil and more unsaturated ("good") fat or oil.

Not all fats and oils are harmful. Some of them *raise* your blood cholesterol level; others actually *lower* it. Knowing how to tell the difference allows you to cut back on the "bad," or saturated, fats and replace them with "good," or unsaturated, ones. This is the main key to painless cholesterol control.

STEP ONE: Distinguish saturated from unsaturated fats as groundwork for an artery-sparing diet. Saturated fats push your cholesterol *up*. "Saturated" has nothing to do with moisture; it's a chemical term that means that the fat molecules have all the hydrogen atoms they can possibly hold. This includes most fats that stay firm at room temperature, for example, lard, suet, Crisco®, butter, cocoa butter, and chicken fat. (Margarine is the main exception.) It also includes most of the oils used commercially, either in restaurant frying or in prepared salad dressings and the like, such as palm kernel oil, palm oil, and coconut oil.

Most of the cooking oils you buy in your grocery store are *unsaturated*. Corn oil (e.g., Mazola®), cottonseed oil (e.g.,

---

"Bad" (Saturated) Fats

Coconut oil	Pork fat (lard)
Cocoa butter (chocolate)	Chicken fat
Palm oil	Turkey fat
Butterfat	Bacon drippings
Beef fat (tallow)	

Wesson®), canola oil (e.g., Puritan®), olive oil, sunflower oil, safflower oil, and peanut oil *help* your arteries instead of *hurt* them. Your arteries benefit two ways when you substitute "good" for "bad":

- Each percentage point *decrease* in "bad" fat lowers your blood cholesterol three units.
- Each percentage point *increase* in "good" fat lowers your blood cholesterol one-and-a-half units.[2]

If you're like me, you have a limited store of willpower, so it makes sense to use what you've got where it will do the most good. That's mainly in the kitchen instead of at the dining table! Of the fat or oil you consume, less than one-fifth is table fat—butter for your bread, sour cream for your potato, and the like. The rest—*four times as much*—comes from ingredients you use in your cooking.

STEP TWO: Get double benefits by replacing the "bad" fats with "good" ones in cooking. This approach gets top billing for two reasons:

- It involves almost no sacrifice.
- You get double the benefit. *Less* saturated fat pushes down your blood cholesterol. *More* unsaturated fat pushes it down even further!

"Good" (Unsaturated) Fats

Canola oil (Puritan®)	Soybean oil
Safflower oil	Cottonseed oil (Wesson®)
Sunflower oil	Peanut oil
Corn oil (Mazola®)	Margarine
Olive oil	

---

[2] Peter Kwiterovich, M.D., *Beyond Cholesterol* (The Johns Hopkins University Press, Baltimore & London, 1989), p.176.

Anything you now fry in butter will taste just as good if you use margarine. You can also use olive oil or Puritan® for frying along with some oil-soluble herbs such as thyme, marjoram, and rosemary. Making your own salad dressings, barbecue sauce, meat sauce, and dip to replace commercial ones that have a lot of saturated fat actually improves the flavor in most cases.

You'll find that most recipes from standard cookbooks either already use unsaturated fats and oils or can be adapted just by substituting an equal amount of unsaturated fat or oil for the saturated, or "bad," fat.

It's a bit harder to adapt baking recipes, so I've put three basic ones in boxes scattered throughout the next few pages. You'll find recipes for

- A basic cookie with several optional variations
- A spice cake (spices obscure the difference in flavor between butter and margarine) to which a variety of fruits can be added for variation
- A pie crust that requires no rolling out and various fillings

All these baked goods freeze well, so you can make worthwhile quantities while you're at it.

Perhaps you won't always have to give up ready-prepared salad dressings, sauces, and dips or even baked goods. While most of those on the market today use "bad" tropical oils, recently a few food companies have introduced products with canola or olive oil. New Food and Drug Administration regulations also make labels less deceptive, easier to read, and more understandable, so as food companies make more healthful products, you'll be able to identify and use them.

STEP THREE: Confine butter to the table only. This takes us to the issue of dairy products. Should you use some of your remaining willpower to replace butter with margarine? It depends on how great a sacrifice doing so would be for *you*. My wife and I cannot abide using margarine as a spread for biscuits or vegetables, so we use margarine in cooking, but not at the table. Many of our friends, on the other hand, hardly notice the difference between these spreads. Others find a blend satisfactory.

Raisin or Fruited Spice Cake

Preheat oven to 325°F.

1 cup beer	1/8 teaspoonful nutmeg
1 cup brown sugar	2 cups of seeded raisins or
1/3 cup margarine	chopped dry figs or
1/2 teaspoonful cinnamon	chopped pecans or
1/2 teaspoonful allspice	chopped dry apricots or
1/2 teaspoonful salt	chopped dates

Combine ingredients and boil for 3 minutes. Let cool.

2 cups cake flour	1 teaspoonful baking soda
1 teaspoonful double-acting baking powder	1 cup chopped almonds

Sift cake flour. Resift with baking powder and baking soda. Stir flour gradually into other ingredients. Stir batter until smooth. Add almonds. Bake in a greased 7-inch tube pan for 1 hour or more.

Make icing by beating with a wire whisk 2 egg whites, 1/2 cup sugar, and 2 tablespoonfuls cold water until blended. Place in double boiler over boiling water. Beat for 3 minutes or until stiff. Remove from heat. Add 1 teaspoonful vanilla extract. Beat well, then spread on cake.

If giving up butter at the table is a real sacrifice for you, don't do it! You can accomplish much more with less impact on your life-style by saving willpower for the measures already described. But butter *as an ingredient* is another matter.

You can accomplish a lot toward sparing your arteries by never using butter in the kitchen. You'll hardly miss it if you make these three simple substitutions:

- Fry, braise, and broil with margarine or olive oil instead of butter.

- Replace high-fat cheeses like cheddar and Swiss with low-fat ones. Edam, Gouda, Fontina, Fontinella, and any other cheeses labeled "made from whole (or partly skimmed) milk" taste great without the extra butterfat. You can also use strongly flavored cheeses like Parmesan or Romano. These have lots of fat per ounce, but their intense flavor makes a little bit go a long way.

- Try frozen yoghurt instead of ice cream. You can cut out the equivalent of four or five pats of butter per serving!

STEP FOUR: Cut down on "bad" fats. You also help keep your arteries supple simply by *cutting down* on saturated fats. You can do this with only a little more impact on your life-style than substitution if you separate out animal fat, almost all of which is saturated, and leave it in the kitchen.

- Instead of frying or panbroiling, grill meats so that the fat drains away.

- Keep two stockpots in the refrigerator, one for juices from red meat and one for juices from poultry. Before you add each ration of meat juice, refrigerate it in a separate container. Remove the fat after it rises to the top and solidifies. Add the remaining fluid to your stockpot. Use fat-free stock to make gravy, sauces, and soups. Save fresh meat juice and defat it to replenish your supply.

Next come the only things you do at the table instead of in the kitchen:

- Trim off visible fat from beef, veal, pork and ham as you eat it. Although some of the fat in these meats is scattered through the lean portion, it's certainly worthwhile to leave as much as you can on the plate.

- Leave the skin of chicken, turkey, or duck on your plate. Almost all the fat in poultry lies in or just under the skin. Peeling off that layer makes poultry a perfect high-protein, low-fat food.

Crinkle Cookies

3/4 cup margarine
1 cup sugar
1 cup packed brown sugar
2 eggs
1 teaspoonful vanilla
1/4 cup milk
2 cups quick-cooking rolled oats

1 (4 oz.) package salted sunflower seeds
2 cups flour
1/2 teaspoonful baking powder
1 teaspoonful baking soda
1/4 teaspoonful salt

Plus any two of the following:

1 cup flake coconut
1 cup raisins
1 cup dried bananas
1 cup chopped citron

1 cup chopped walnuts
1 cup chopped pecans
1 cup cranberries
1 cup chopped dry apricots

Preheat oven to 350°F. Cream margarine and sugars. Beat in eggs, vanilla, and milk. Combine flour, baking powder, baking soda, salt, and oats. Blend into creamed mixture until moistened. Stir in sunflower seeds and the two optional ingredients you have chosen. Drop by rounded teaspoonfuls onto greased baking sheets. Bake until edges are browned, 13 to 15 minutes. Be sure to leave on baking sheets until firm and cool. Makes about 4 dozen.

- Eat lots of fish and shellfish, which have little or no saturated fat. (Don't worry about the cholesterol content of shellfish—the absence of saturated fat more than makes up for it.)

- Trim off the breading or other crispy coating from fried chicken or fish. Almost all the added "bad" fat in commercially fried chicken or fish stays in the surface coating as long as the fryer stays up to temperature. If you avoid "rush hour" (when heavy use often drops the cooking temperature so that more fat absorbs into the meat itself) and trim off the coating with the skin, even fast food chicken won't poison your arteries.

At only forty-one, Nancy O. was definitely headed for artery trouble. Both her parents had heart attacks before they were fifty, and her grandfather had had a stroke. Nancy's examination and lab tests showed further reasons to worry:

- *Her eyelids had several little yellowish raised plaques, which often indicate high cholesterol.*

- *Her blood studies showed a reading of 260—well above the 200 "top of normal."*

When I explained saturated and unsaturated fats and oils to Nancy, she balked at changing her recipes. She said "I really don't want to fix all my own meals separately from the family's" or "put my kids on a special diet just because I need one."

The health teacher at her youngsters' high school finally did more to convince her than I. A display at the science fair showed how the roots of arteriosclerosis trace back to your teens—hamburgers, French fries, and milkshakes start a lot of scales inside your arteries. When Nancy realized that she would be doing her whole family a favor by feeding all of them according to my recommendations, she did. She began making her own salad dressing with olive oil, serving ham and pastrami made from turkey instead of pork or beef, and substituting canola oil for butter in her spice cookies. To her surprise, both her husband and her children not only ate the new dishes but complimented her on them.

A few months later, Nancy's blood cholesterol had dropped to 185. That was ten years ago, and Nancy has stayed healthy ever since—even though she's well past the age at which both her parents had heart attacks.

PRIME STRETCHER 3

*Float cholesterol through your artery walls
instead of letting it deposit there.*

Cholesterol can't hurt your arteries if it can't get to them, and it won't dissolve in water or blood. Each molecule needs a "chemical raft" to float on. These rafts lift the cholesterol and carry it through the bloodstream, just as soap dissolves the grease on your dishes.

But some of those rafts do a better job than others. They carry the cholesterol all the way, until your body disposes of it. Those rafts are small and compact, and they go by the name "high-density lipids" or HDL. Small rafts don't get stuck in your artery walls and deteriorate leaving cholesterol behind, as larger ones often do, causing hard plaques. Small rafts even pick up cholesterol that has been deposited in your artery walls and carry it out of plaques that have already formed.

STEP ONE: Build high-density lipids, or HDL, by eating more "good" fat or oil. When you build up your intake of unsaturated fat, you definitely increase your HDL. Since only a few extra units of HDL in your blood can cut your risk of coronary and other arterial disease in half, this can be a big help in stretching your prime. Some specific techniques are

- Fry one extra entree a day in a "good" oil.

- Spread your luncheon sandwiches with a heavy layer of old-fashioned peanut butter.

- Make garlic, onion, chive, or other dips with "good" oil. Eat with small pretzels, Swedish rye wafers, or bread sticks (not high-fat potato chips) as a before-dinner or TV snack.

Since I eat the same breakfast almost every day, I just put olive oil in my frying pan instead of using a spray-on nonstick coating like Pam®. My usual breakfast includes a slice of ham or pastrami made from turkey with one egg, toast,

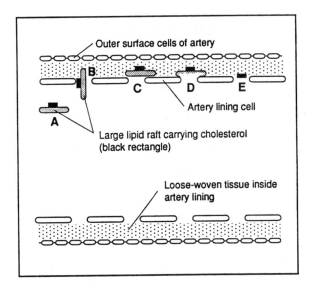

Large floating rafts carrying cholesterol (A) penetrate between loose cells at artery lining (B), get stuck (C), and break down (D), leaving the cholesterol trapped (E).

and jam. I dodge the "butter versus margarine" question by using enough jam that I don't need either.

You might prefer to add your extra "good" oil in the form of salad dressing or margarine. But don't fall for the "all fats are bad" line: "good" fats and oils actually help, both by lowering your blood cholesterol level and by increasing your HDL.

Although eating right probably helps build HDL more than any other approach, several other measures also help.

STEP TWO: Lose excess weight. There are lots of reasons to lose weight, but the fact that it definitely builds HDL might motivate you to make the effort required for getting your weight down *and keeping it* down. This is particularly true if you have had coronary problems, have a family history that suggests that you're prone to heart trouble, or have had blood tests showing either high cholesterol or low HDL.

Pressed-in Pie Crust

Preheat oven to 375°F.

2 tablespoonfuls milk	1½ cups flour
½ cup oil (corn, cottonseed, or canola)	1 teaspoonful salt
	1½ teaspoonful sugar

Whip together milk and oil. Add all at once to flour mixture. Mix with a fork. Press into pie pan, prick, and bake for 15 minutes. Use apple, berry, cherry, raisin, mince, or pecan filling (without whipped cream).

STEP THREE: Stop smoking. If you haven't already done so (shame on you!), this step will add about 5 HDL units—enough to cut your coronary risk more than in half. (See page 294 for help.)

STEP FOUR: Exercise regularly. Chapters 2 and 12 give specific suggestions for regular exercise. Just remember that more people *rust* out than *wear* out—the rocking chair and davenport may have more hazards than the track! Activity *builds* HDL, inactivity *erodes* it!

PRIME STRETCHER 4

Help your arteries further with blood thinners.

Your blood contains chemical glues as well as chemical rafts. These chemical glues help when you have an injury by sticking various elements together into a clot. But they also play a part in trapping cholesterol-carrying rafts in your artery walls.

Blood thinners protect your arteries by cutting down these floating gluelike enzymes. Although this also makes your blood clot less readily (which is a disadvantage), it gives your arteries tremendous help. Less stickiness lets even large chemical rafts pass through your artery lining without getting stuck and helps small rafts carry away some of the cholesterol that is already there.

STEP ONE: Use aspirin as a blood thinner. *Small amounts* of aspirin block the formation of the clot-forming glue (which also causes cholesterol-carrying rafts to stick in your vessel walls). Larger doses cancel out this effect. They block the formation of another body substance that normally fights the glue's effects. (Your body often uses substances with opposite action in balance against one another to regulate its more delicate processes.)

If you use aspirin to protect your arteries, you need to follow two rules:

- *Do* take half an adult-size (5-grain) aspirin every single day. To keep your body from forming these floating glue-like enzymes, you need active agents constantly in your system. You can't make up for gaps in coverage because there's no way to remove the enzyme (until it wears out naturally) once you've let it form.

- *Don't* take more aspirin for *any* reason. Control headaches, joint pains, and so on with agents that have a completely different mechanism of action like ibuprofen (the less expensive generic form of Advil® or Motrin®).

A great many doctors (including me) take aspirin every day for this purpose. But remember that the same lack of glue that makes cholesterol-carrying rafts slide through your vessel walls more easily also makes your blood clot more slowly, which is a real drawback. If you follow this program, your blood vessels will not seal leaks as rapidly as they should. For instance, I cut myself the other day. It wasn't much of a cut, but I had to keep pressure on it for 20 minutes before it stopped bleeding.

You shouldn't use aspirin if you need to keep your blood's clotting ability totally up to snuff, for example, if you've had a stomach ulcer that might bleed internally. If you have any injury that involves broken or cut blood vessels while you are taking aspirin, you should use ice and local pressure for longer than usual to control bleeding (or bruising, which is bleeding under the skin). *If you get any sign of internal bleeding—soft stools black as tar, vomiting blood, or light headedness with rapid pulse—call your doctor right away.* You're not likely to have such trouble, or all of us doctors who take aspirin daily wouldn't take the risk. But if you're the rare, unlucky one, you'll need immediate help.

STEP TWO: Use fish oils as an alternate or additional way to thin your blood. When doctors learned of the relationship between dietary fat and arteriosclerosis, they came upon one exception: Eskimos. Eskimos eat enormous amounts of fat. But they have very little arterial disease.

Lots of the fat Eskimos eat comes from whale and seal blubber, which is unsaturated. But the gluelike clotting factors just discussed also play a part. Early Arctic explorers noted that Eskimos not only almost never had heart attacks, they also didn't form normal clots when injured, and their blood remained abnormally liquid for hours after death.

We know now that an acid found in *fish oils* causes such changes in the blood. Certain fish oils have such an intense effect that they even help remove established arteriosclerotic plaques. For instance, scientists can treat pigs in such a way that they form huge arteriosclerotic plaques. But an ounce of cod liver oil a day keeps similarly treated pigs' arteries completely supple.

Cod liver oil also seems to work for people, although that's harder to prove. But a more pleasant way to get fish oil is to eat fish! Four ounces of salmon supplies more of the key blood-thinning substance than seven fish oil acid capsules[3], which are the main alternative and work well if you don't want to eat a lot of seafood.

---

[3] Available products include Promega®, GNC mega-EPA 1000®, Royal Oak epa Plus® and Solgan MaxEPA®.

GOOD SOURCES OF FISH OIL		
Rich Sources of Fish Oil		**Less Rich Sources of Fish Oil**
Shellfish	*Oily Finfish*	*Less Oily Finfish*
King crab	Anchovy	Bass, fresh water
Blue crab	Bluefish	Bass, striped
Lobster	Herring	Cod
Shrimp	Mackerel	Flounder
Clam	Salmon	Haddock
Mussel	Lake trout	Rainbow trout
Oyster	Whitefish	Snapper
Scallop	Tuna	Shark

Fish oil acid works very much the same way as aspirin. You don't usually need to use *both*, just one or the other.

I use aspirin instead of fish oil myself for several reasons. The extra ounce or more of fat intake per day in fish oil means I would have to cut down on calorie intake elsewhere, and I really enjoy my food. Also, you need a healthy gallbladder to digest all that oil. But fish oil (or its key acid) certainly is worthwhile for people who can't take aspirin (because of allergy or stomach ulcers). You may also want to give it a try if your family history, weight, blood pressure, or smoking habit makes you highly prone to coronary or other arterial disorders. And it seems worth a try if you need to remove already-deposited plaques.

HOW HARD SHOULD YOU WORK
AT ARTERY SPARING?

The following table will help you decide how intense a program you should follow.

If you're a young woman whose parents and grandparents have had no coronaries or strokes, your arteries will probably stay in good shape regardless. But substituting unsaturated for saturated fats doesn't cost a cent or hurt a thing. So why not take out a little extra insurance?

Your hormones give you less protection after the menopause, and some extra measures become worthwhile.

Even with a good family history, men have more coronary risk. Adding aspirin to your program cuts that risk in half.

Extra risk factors certainly make it worthwhile to limit saturated fat. You should keep dietary cholesterol (mainly eggs) at a reasonable level without going to extreme measures.

With a known and established problem, go all out. Include fish oil in your diet if you can keep your weight down and don't get indigestion from it.

FACTORS TO CONSIDER IN CHOOSING APT SCLEROSIS-FIGHTING MEASURES

Your Situation	Substitute Unsaturated Fat	Limit Saturated Fat	Aspirin	Fish Oil	Cut Cholesterol
Premenopausal woman, good genes	X				
Postmenopausal woman, good genes	X		X		
Man, good genes	X		X	*	
Smoker, or 20% overweight, or coronaries, strokes, in family	X	X	X	*	One less egg daily
Coronary or arteriosclerotic disease, known high blood cholesterol	X	X	X	X	Follow prescribed diet

*If you can't take aspirin

CHAPTER 2

Circulation Boosters

When you talk about "losing your circulation," you're probably thinking "cold hands and feet." That's the most obvious result of the sluggish blood flow caused by advancing age. You need circulation to bring warmth to your extremities. But you also need it to bring oxygen to your brain and muscles. And you need it to empty veins as well as fill arteries.

Chapter 2 offers you five ways to keep aging at bay with improved circulation:

- Keeping warm blood on the move
- Exercising to open up partly clogged leg arteries
- Keeping your heart in shape with exercise
- Warding off stroke
- Avoiding congestion in your veins

PRIME STRETCHER 1

*Keep warm blood flowing through your
fingers and toes.*

Your body is generally surrounded with cool air. Heat flows from the inside through your skin into that cool air. To stay warm, each body part has to *gain* as much heat from circulating warm blood as it *loses* through its surface. Body parts like your fingers, toes, and ears have very little heat-retaining bulk, a lot of exposed surface through which to lose heat, and only a few small blood vessels through which to gain warm blood flow.

STEP ONE: Keep fingers and toes warm by wearing a hat or cap (even indoors). Your body has a way of preserving heat that robs fingers and toes of warmth-giving circulation. When your brain and inner organs need warmth, your system preserves it by short-circuiting the blood that's going toward your fingers and toes. Special passages in your wrists and ankles open up and take most of the warm blood that would normally go through your fingers and toes directly from approaching arteries to nearby veins, which take it back to your brain and inner organs while it is still warm. Your fingers and toes get just enough circulation to stay alive, not enough to stay comfortable.

The most important single step you can take to maintain general body warmth is to cut heat loss from your scalp. Your scalp gets its blood from the same vessels that supply your brain. All circulation control systems work to make sure your brain gets adequate blood flow, so those vessels never close off no matter how cold you get. While the vessels to the rest of your skin have squeezed down to save body heat, those to your scalp stay wide open. That fact, plus the vast number of blood vessels in the scalp (which you'll appreciate if you've ever seen how even a small scalp wound bleeds), means that almost one-third of your body's heat loss comes from your eyebrows up.

You can see why wearing a hat will preserve body heat so that your system won't cut off warm blood intended for your fingers and toes. If you have trouble with cold fingers or toes, get at least two pieces of warm head wear, one suitable for indoor wear (perhaps a knitted cap, skullcap, or beret) and one for outdoor wear. Wear them constantly for a day or two and see what they do for your problem. Then you may even go for a coonskin cap or a nightcap—those pioneers weren't so dumb!

STEP TWO: Insulate the rest of your body, too. Although your scalp accounts for over 30 percent of your body's heat loss, that still leaves 70 percent dissipating elsewhere. Clothing chosen for style instead of warmth still limits this loss to some degree, but often not sufficiently to keep your blood thoroughly warm.

Heavier undergarments help. Long johns or snuggies do as much to keep your fingers warm as mittens by keeping your blood warm and reducing the need for short-circuiting blood destined for your extremities. Wool sweaters, jackets, and skirts also help. Synthetics may seem to have the same texture, but they just don't keep you as warm.

Grace A.'s experience shows just how well limiting heat loss from the scalp and body works in warming cold fingers and toes. Grace came to my office the first time on a mild spring day, but wearing mittens and galoshes. When I asked about these, she told me that her fingers and toes stayed just like ice, even at home with the heat turned fairly high.

Grace's other clothing was more stylish than warm. Her cotton print dress had a deep V neck, she didn't wear a hat, and the coat she carried had more sheen than thickness. I explained to her the need for whole body (and especially scalp) warmth. At first she didn't believe that wearing a warm hat had anything to do with keeping her hands and feet warm, so I asked my wife to loan her a knitted cap and a down vest for a few days. Grace tried wearing them in her own home (they did look pretty strange!) and became convinced. When she returned my wife's head and body warmers, she had on a warm hat, sweater, and wool slacks of her own, which she reported were totally effective in keeping her feet and fingers warm.

PRIME STRETCHER 2

*Open up narrowing leg arteries with
Buerger-Allen exercises.*

If circulation to your legs becomes so sluggish that your legs
remain cold even when your trunk and scalp are warm, narrowed
arteries probably are at fault.

**STEP ONE: Identify poor arterial circulation to make Buer-
ger-Allen exercises worthwhile.** Buerger-Allen exercises take
time to complete, and sometimes as much as three months to
begin to help. So you don't want to start them unless you're
fairly sure you need them.

If your leg arteries are narrowed, your legs will actually
feel cold to your touch and look somewhat pale. As the limited
circulation increases, you may find that you get cramps in the
muscles when you walk a long way.[1] Cramps due to poor
arterial circulation feel like a hot iron pressing into your muscle
rather than like an ordinary cramp, and often aren't accompanied
by the knotting up of the muscle, which occurs with other
types of cramps. They generally occur very predictably after
a certain amount of exercise: if a cramp occurs one day after
you've walked five blocks, you'll seldom be able to walk much
farther than that the next day without getting a similar cramp.

If cramps come on with only moderate exertion—a half-mile
walk or less—or if you have any reason to suspect that you
are extra prone to hardened arteries (e.g., diabetes or a family
history of artereosclerotic disease), you should check with your
doctor right away. Vascular surgery has come a long way,
and the plaques that narrow arteries can often be removed to
restore circulation completely. For milder conditions (for which
you wouldn't even consider surgery), do these exercises three
times a day:

---

[1] See also page 37 for discussion of other types of leg cramps.

1. Turn a straight chair over on the lower half of your bed, so that the legs of the chair stick out over the foot of the bed and the chair's back forms an angled platform for your legs when you lie down. Pad the back of the chair with a folded sheet or blanket. Lie on your back with your legs stretched along the inclined chair back. Remain in this position for 2 minutes.

2. Sit up with your feet dangling over the side of the bed. Slowly and deliberately carry out each possible foot and toe motion: turn your toes down, raise them up, turn your feet inward, turn them outward, spread your toes, curl them and raise them.

3. Lie flat on the bed with your feet and legs wrapped in warm blankets. Relax in this position for 5 minutes.

These exercises stretch the tiny blood vessels that have the most resistance to blood flow. As I said, this is a very gradual process, though. So don't lose patience!

PRIME STRETCHER 3

Use physical activity to help heart health.

"Use it or lose it" applies very strongly to your physical reserve. You need physical activity to maintain heart strength, which helps you to stretch your prime and hold aging at bay. This is almost always true even if you've had a heart attack or other heart disease (although you should check with your doctor in this case to be sure).

A totally sedentary life ages your heart fast. Just being on your feet and walking an hour a day vastly decreases your chance of getting heart and circulatory problems. A higher level of activity gives you an even better chance of avoiding such difficulties.

Even if you're quite active now, that doesn't mean you'll never need these techniques. Some time in the future an injury, illness, or change in circumstances may interrupt your sports or exercise program. That's how so many people get off track, and once their activity pattern is interrupted, a vicious circle begins. Being out of shape makes it tough to return directly to your previous level, so you remain inactive and get even further out of shape. You need a concrete method of resuming activity after any interruption.

If you've already been caught in that web (or weren't very active in the first place), here's how to get in gear.

STEP ONE: Learn to count your pulse so that you can tell how much exercise you can safely do as you get back into condition. When your system burns enough fuel that it needs extra oxygen, your body stretches its capacities to meet that need. Each "stretch" builds a bit of extra heart-lung power (until you reach your maximum, which happens only if you push yourself to the limit). When you are out of shape, the only activities that help you get back into condition are aerobic ones: those that call on your body's reserves.

Activities don't need to be strenuous to be aerobic. They generally involve continual use of a substantial portion of your muscle mass: body and leg muscles are much larger than arm muscles, so their contraction uses considerable fuel and increases oxygen demand. Walking, bicycling, rowing, swimming, and cross-country skiing all accomplish this goal as do more strenuous activities such as running or lifting weights.

The best way to tell whether an activity is stretching your capacities is to count your pulse. If you don't already know how to do this, here's a simple technique:

1. Wear a wristwatch on your left arm so that you can see it easily while you feel the artery in your right wrist.

2. Turn your right-hand palm up. Lay your left index, middle and ring fingers in a row between the thumbside wrist bone and the wrist's bundle of tendons. You'll feel the pulse beat with one or more fingers.

3. Count for 15 seconds and multiply by four. If you check your pulse before you exercise, you can recheck as a way of pacing yourself.

4. Count your pulse at intervals as you exercise. Whenever it has increased, you've done enough to improve your heart-lung condition. You can safely continue (if you feel like it) until your pulse has increased twenty beats per minute beyond its resting level. At that point, you've stretched yourself far enough. Doing more does no further good, so rest until your count goes down before continuing.

STEP TWO: Choose activities you can perform frequently. If you exercise any muscle adequately, including your heart muscle, you increase its strength. That increase tapers gradually

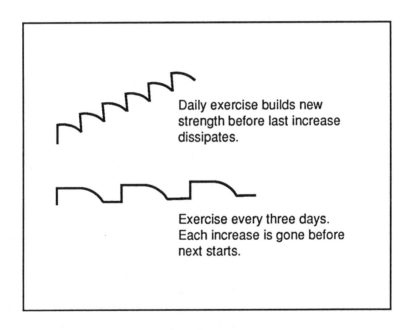

Frequent exercise builds strength by adding new increments on top of the old. Infrequent exercise leaves strength largely unchanged.

over a period of about two days. If you exercise it adequately again within that period of time, you build further strength on top of that already developed. If you wait until the previous increase has disappeared, increases in strength don't enhance one another: instead of a curve that looks like a stairway, you get bumps on a level line (see illustration). Set aside time for physical activity at least three or four times a week. *Often* is better than *hard* or *long*!

When getting into shape, it's important to choose activities you can perform frequently, but it isn't necessary to do the same thing every time. You can swim on the days the school pool is available to adults, walk on sunny days and use a rowing machine when it rains, for instance. The key is to have alternatives that suit all kinds of weather and circumstances, so that you never go more than two days without exercise.

STEP THREE: Emphasize activities that you can readily quantify. Pick noncompetitive, steady-action exercises like walking, bicycling, rowing, or swimming. (We'll talk more about sports and games in Chapter 12. They're great once you're in shape, but to get started you need continuous mild exertion. Most sports involve spurts of action with long pauses between.) Until you get into reasonably good shape, you need to let your conditioning requirements and state govern the intensity and duration of activity. Any time you're trying to win, to perform up to standard, or even to put in a good showing, you're likely to overdo, to get discouraged, or both. Let pulse changes and symptoms rather than competitive pressures tell you how far to go.

Not that every change in the way you feel should make you quit. Don't worry if you become slightly short of breath or weak during an activity. You can continue to exercise if these sensations remain mild. If you feel tightness or mild discomfort in your chest, slow down until those feelings abate, but don't let them frighten you or make you quit. Those symptoms warn you to slow down before you do yourself any harm. (Heart specialists tell their recovering coronary patients to push activity right up to the point of pain. Forget about heart trouble dooming you to the rocking chair!)

When you're first trying to get into shape, always plan ahead to provide for any rest breaks you might need. When I was getting back on my feet after having surgery for cancer, I carried a "shooting stick"—a cane with a handle that turns into a seat—on my walks. If I started to get tired, I would perch on the shooting stick and watch the birds (or the people) for a while. Some of my patients take their first few walks in a park where there are lots of benches. Others trade in variety for extra security and go round and round their home block, so that they can rest if necessary. All these approaches beat starting around the lake when you might get tired on the other side.

Build a little at a time. Walk around the block, then around two blocks, then around three. Seeing progress will help keep you at it. Work up to a brisk 20-minute walk, bike ride or swim before you try games or sports, even among friends who won't be upset if you quit. (Your desire to keep up with the crowd might still make you overdo.)

Harry P. had always been able almost to chase me off the tennis court. At fifty-five, he used to warm up for the game by jogging a mile or so. Then he dropped out of sight for a while.

When I met him on the street one day he explained what had happened. First, he had torn a muscle in his leg, which took three months to heal. Then, before he got back into action, he came back from Mexico with the tourista, which lasted for about a month. When he finally got back to the courts, he found that he had "just plain lost it." His heart started pounding as soon as he ran after a few balls. He felt worn out after a few games, long before the match ended.

At this point, Harry figured that he was "just past it." He thought that his body was telling him something—that he couldn't keep on forever, and at nearly sixty it was time to quit.

Harry had hit a very common snag. He had gotten out of shape from injury and illness. He couldn't jump back into action at the old level, so he just gave up.

When all this came out during our conversation, I protested. I explained to Harry that he could almost certainly get back into action if he went about it gradually instead of leaping right into the fray. Then I mailed him a sheet explaining how to rebuild circulation, which outlined exactly the steps I've just explained. About a month later, Harry showed up on the tennis court again and he was back in top form. Beat me 6–4, 6–3!

PRIME STRETCHER 4

Build heart attack–preventing HDL with exercise.

Exercise works almost as well as a rigid diet in building high density lipids (HDL), the small cholesterol-carrying rafts in your blood that help keep your arteries supple. Just a few extra units of this substance can cut your heart attack risk in half! These measures can readily provide them:

1. Get back in shape with Prime Stretcher 2 if necessary.

2. Keep track for a few days to see how much exercise you get through your usual routines. Whenever you walk any distance, climb stairs, do household chores, or do any big-muscle activity, check your pulse rate (see page 24). Anything that raises your pulse rate eight beats or more is an HDL builder.

3. Unless you're getting at least one hour of pulse-raising exercise a day, fill in the gaps with brisk walks.

Peter G. gave me a chance to check what exercise could do for one's HDL. After recovering from a heart attack, Peter followed a rigid low-cholesterol, low-fat diet to the letter. But his blood tests still showed a dangerous lack of high-density lipids. In spite of what his cardiologist and I had told him, he remained afraid that exercise might bring on another heart attack.

I reassured him again and again, and finally convinced him that exercise was more likely to ward off than to bring on another attack.

"Exercise changes your body chemistry," I explained. "It increases your HDL, which washes cholesterol out of your arteries and makes the obstructing plaques actually shrink."

Peter decided on walking as the easiest exercise to arrange and built up to brisk half-hour walks every day. Three months later, his blood tests showed a five-unit increase in HDL. That one change meant that he had cut his chance of another heart attack in half! Quite a reward for walking a few hours a week, when he had made absolutely no other changes in his life-style!

PRIME STRETCHER 5

Use vigorous physical activity to develop extra blood flow passages within your heart muscle.

We've all heard about people who dropped dead on the tennis court. You hear about such events over and over because they are remarkable enough to be "news." Actually, you should be much more afraid of the couch than the playing field.

STEP ONE: Use vigorous exercise to build heart health once you are in reasonable shape. Sudden death happens about ten times as often per hour during rest as during exertion. Vigorous exercise not only *prevents* many heart attacks by building HDL, it also *makes any attacks that do occur much milder* by getting your coronary arteries to expand. The coronary passages get larger to handle exertion's peak loads. Since these vessels interconnect at many points, they provide detours around any point at which blockage might later occur.

Don't let either fear or sloth rob you of these benefits. Unless arthritis or other health problems limit you severely, either

- Pick a vigorous sport and stick with it (see Chapter 12) or

- Consider jogging.

STEP TWO: See whether jogging is right for you. Most people think of jogging as exercise for the sake of fitness. That's how it usually starts, but it often turns into something more than that.

"There's nothing like it," one of my patients said. "After you run for a while, you get this feeling that you could go forever. It's like you're treading on air, and nothing in the world matters."

That's runner's high, a country cousin of second wind. People who stick with jogging or running almost always report this phenomenon. They inevitably run just far enough to enjoy it for a while. If they get second wind in half a mile, they run a mile and quit. If they have to run three miles to get it, their normal workout goes at least four.

When you get into either second wind or runner's high, your brain waves look exactly as if you're hypnotized. This puts runner's high in the same category as transcendental meditation, autoconditioning, self-hypnosis, and yoga. If you can achieve this condition, it will do a lot for you both physically and mentally. Besides long-range effects on your HDL and coronary arteries, your exercise brings an instant reward—it lifts your mood and eases your tensions. That's enough to keep you coming back without using up your willpower.

Will you definitely experience that feeling? You'll never know unless you try. But if you *do* try, follow these rules:

- Get good footwear. Jogging shoes should cushion the impact of your feet with the ground so that transmitted thumps don't jar your knees.

- Choose a smooth course. Running on rough or uneven ground can harm your joints.

- Pick dull surroundings, or ignore their points of interest. Concentrate on the soothing, hypnotic rhythm of your steps. (Most veteran joggers stare straight ahead and ultimately get a glazed look that coincides with their "high.")

- While building capacity, check your pulse at intervals. If it goes over 140, walk until it drops below 100, then jog again.

- Ask an experienced runner, coach, or physiotherapist to help you with your posture, stride, and arm movements. If you can improve body dynamics, you'll keep down the wear and tear on joints, which is jogging's main drawback.

When you ask a medical specialist about jogging, it's like asking a blind man to describe an elephant. His answer will depend on what part of your body he usually checks. The heart people say "great," while the bone people shake their heads.

Here's my advice: If you want to try it, follow the rules just given and build up to at least a two-mile run. If you're getting a second wind or runner's high, you'll keep with it. Otherwise, you'll be better off looking for another sport (which you'll almost automatically do; almost nobody keeps jogging on the basis of self-discipline alone).

PRIME STRETCHER 6

*Ward off strokes with blood pressure
control, aspirin, and Persantine®.*

Strokes seldom happen with no detectable warning. Detectable high
blood pressure precedes many of them. Brief malfunctions called
TIAs—transient (brief) ischemic (lack of blood supply) attacks—
warn of others. Prompt treatment of these premonitors staves off
most strokes and preserves crucial functions through the years.

**STEP ONE: Check your own blood pressure at intervals to
help prevent stroke and heart failure.** The easiest way to
check your blood pressure is with the machines found in most
drugstores. These machines generally give an accurate reading
if the cuff wraps snugly around your arm and if your upper
arm's girth is 10 inches or less. A loosely wrapped cuff or
one too small for your arm gives a false reading, usually about
10 millimeters (mm.) high. I'll explain why in a moment. These
machines are fully automatic and give a digital readout, so
you don't need instructions in their use.

  If you have never had high blood pressure readings, get
a reading every three months or so. As long as the upper
reading is under 140 mm. and the lower reading is below 90
mm., don't worry about your blood pressure. In particular don't
worry about *low* readings. If the high reading is under 100
mm., you may occasionally get dizzy if you stand up too suddenly,
but you'll outlive most people with average readings and have
almost no risk of stroke.

  Chances are that if you are headed for high blood pressure,
you will get a few temporarily high readings. Your doctor will
take your pressure, then chat with you a few minutes, and
take it again. Then he'll tell you that you may have been a
little excited the first time, but the initially high reading came
down to normal later.

  If this happens, you don't need blood pressure treatment,
but you should get proper equipment and learn to take your own
pressure. You'll accomplish three worthwhile goals in this way:

- You'll find readings at home reassuring. No matter how comfortable you feel with your doctor, your pressure generally goes up when he wraps that cuff around your arm. Back home you may still find the first few checks mildly upsetting, but you can take repeat readings until they settle down. After a while the whole procedure becomes so routine that it doesn't excite you any longer. Your pressure taken under ordinary circumstances is the most accurate, not readings taken during upsetting doctor visits.

- If your pressure does become abnormal, you'll detect it promptly. With dozens of different medicines available these days, you and your doctor can almost surely find one that controls your pressure without major side effects.

- Equally important, you can *keep from getting started on blood pressure medicines you don't need.* Once you get a few high or borderline readings, it gets harder and harder to relax while your doctor is taking your pressure. Unless he's very patient, he'll take two or three readings and then assume the last one (even if it's still high) was accurate. He'll then start you on blood pressure medicine, and when you come in next time with lower readings (whether from the medicine or just because you're more at ease by then), he'll say that you're doing great so why change a winning game? You can prevent this very common succession of events by knowing what your *right* readings are—because your reasonably skilled readings at home *are* more likely to be more accurate than even highly skilled readings under emotionally upsetting circumstances.

You can get equipment with the right size cuff ("Standard" if your arm measures 10 inches or less, "Wide" if your arm is larger) of either the automatic or the ordinary type. Because automatic units give digital readouts, all you need to do is wrap the cuff snugly and follow directions. If you use the substantially less expensive dial readout type, follow these directions:

1. With your left arm slightly bent flex its biceps muscle. This makes its tendon at the elbow stand up tight so that you can easily feel it. The main artery in your arm lies just toward the inner side of your arm from that tendon. Note this spot and remember where it is.

2. Sit in an armchair. Wrap the cuff snugly and smoothly around your upper arm with the center of its rubber balloon above the artery. (Some cuffs have an arrow that should be placed over the artery's location.) If the cuff has a built-in stethoscope, be sure that its end is located over the artery. Otherwise, use an un-attached stethoscope to listen over that area.

3. Hold your arm out straight with its weight supported at the elbow by the arm of the chair. Clip the dial attached to the cuff to its surface so that you can easily read the numbers. When you first take your pressure, close the valve (adjacent to the squeeze bulb with which you pump air into the cuff). Pump up the cuff until the dial reads 200. The cuff will squeeze your arm rather uncomfortably, which is unavoidable. (After you know the approximate level of your pressure, you can usually pump up the cuff until the dial reads 20 units or so above your last reading, avoiding this discomfort.)

4. Adjust the valve so that air escapes slowly from the cuff, allowing the pressure to drop gradually. Listen carefully with the stethoscope. As the pressure drops, it will reach a point at which you hear a ticking sound with each heartbeat. This indicates that the artery is opening and closing with each pulse wave (you hear the snap as it closes). That means that the pressure inside the artery is rising above that in the cuff at the peak of the pulse wave. Read the dial at this point. This number is your *systolic* blood pressure—the highest pressure exerted on the inside of the vessel.

5. Continue to let air escape gradually so that the pressure inside the cuff falls further. The sounds you hear will modify into a swoosh. When the sound disappears altogether, that means the pressure inside the vessel is higher than that in the cuff throughout the pulse wave. Read the dial at that point. That number indicates your *diastolic* pressure, the pressure that persists through-out the pulse wave.

Blood pressure readings are customarily written like a fraction, with the systolic reading above the line and the diastolic below. An average reading is about 120/80—120 units systolic, 80 units diastolic. You should take readings every 2 minutes until you get three or more readings that are within four units of each other. Ignore the earlier readings and consider only the last three. Your final systolic readings should be below 140 and your diastolic ones below 90. If either reading is too high, check with your doctor. (The diastolic reading is more important, since it indicates the pressure being exerted on vessel walls during most of the pulse cycle. If it is consistently above 90, treatment is almost always worthwhile, and your ability to take readings at home will help your doctor determine the minimum dose of medication required. Systolic readings above 140 sometimes indicate readily correctable conditions and deserve medical attention, but may or may not need treatment.)

Keeping your blood pressure within the normal range cuts out a lot of extra wear and tear on your blood vessels. This not only wards off most strokes but also helps keep your heart working well and preserves the health of your arteries. It's a real help to maintaining your prime.

STEP TWO: Take aspirin in the same doses recommended in Chapter 1 for sparing your arteries. While a few strokes come from a burst blood vessel, the vast majority come from a stopped-up one. Exactly the same approach that keeps clots from clogging up your coronary arteries also keeps clots from clogging up arteries to portions of your brain. Artery-sparing aspirin doses (see page 13) cut your chance of having a stroke almost as much as they reduce your chance of having a heart attack.

STEP THREE: Learn about TIAs so that you can recognize and get treatment for these stroke premonitors. If one of the small arteries in your brain goes into spasm, the nerve cells that are supplied oxygen by that artery cease to function. If the spasm relaxes before a clot forms and makes the stoppage permanent, the interrupted functions resume.

The symptoms you experience when such a spasm occurs vary according to the functions of the oxygen-starved cells.

Even though these complaints may last only a minute or two, you should see a doctor about them promptly. A medication like Persantine® (available only by prescription) will keep further attacks to a minimum and will usually keep the spasm from leading to permanent artery blockage and stroke.

Fifty-two-year-old John F. was watching television when the right half of the screen suddenly went blank. He then found that wherever he looked, he only saw the left half of his normal visual field.

John went to the phone to call me, but by the time the call went through his vision had come back to normal. I had him come in for a checkup and found his blood pressure and other neurologic examination completely normal.

This was a typical TIA, so I asked John to take 25 mg. of Persantine® three times a day. That was 18 years ago. John continues to take the Persantine® as a precaution, but he hasn't had another TIA and has had no sign of stroke.

Common TIA-Caused Complaints

Eye
 Double vision
 Blindness
 Lost vision to either right or left
 Inability to open one eye
Sensations
 Numbness of an arm, leg, side of face, and so on.
 Burning sensation in above areas
Paralysis
 Inability to move half of body, an arm or leg
 Sudden laxness on half of face
Memory Orientation
 Sudden disorientation (not knowing where you are, who you are, the approximate date)

PRIME STRETCHER 7

Control vein congestion with leg vein–draining exercises or external compression.

Many of the circulatory problems you link with aging come from congestion in veins. This can cause swollen feet, leg weariness, painful arches, calf cramps, varicose veins, and skin ulcers on the lower leg.

STEP ONE: Learn how leg muscle contractions pump blood out of your leg veins. You'll avoid leg vein congestion more easily if you understand how the blood normally moves from your legs back to your heart.

The main veins in your leg lie between your calf muscles and the underlying bone. When the muscles contract, they enlarge and squeeze blood out of those veins.

That blood can't travel back into smaller vessels or surface veins because of valves in the vein walls. Those valves work very well as long as the vein remains normal size. Whenever blood tries to flow in the wrong direction, a flap billows away from the vein wall and closes off the passage.

If the vein engorges, the flap no longer reaches all the way across the vein. Blood seesaws back and forth between the deep and surface veins instead of moving on toward the heart. Irritating waste products pile up in the muscles and skin. Bulging surface veins, leg weariness and cramps (from irritating retained waste products), and skin rashes or ulcers result.

STEP TWO: Use support hose to control vein congestion. In the early stages, you can keep veins from becoming so engorged that their valves don't work with these techniques:

- Stand still for 1 minute; then feel for bulging veins in your lower legs. If any feel larger than a lead pencil, wear support hose. The old reliable brand is "Teds®," which you can get fit to your own measurements. You can find them at an orthopedic or hospital supply store. There are some less expensive brands around, too, but be sure they're fit to your own personal measurements rather than being just small, medium, or large.

- As an alternative to support hose, use 4-inch elastic bandages. (A rubberized type like Curity Tensor® or DePuy® works best if rubber doesn't cause your skin to break out. If you're sensitive to rubber, resilient cotton works as long as it keeps its spring, but it tends to lose elasticity and need replacement after a few washings.) Begin with two or three turns on each foot, starting at the base of the toes. You need firm compression of the entire top of your foot to keep fluid from accumulating in the tissues beyond the edge of the bandage. Wrap a figure eight around the ankle twice; then wrap in an overlapping spiral to just below your knee. Fasten the loose end either with the pronged fasteners provided or with adhesive tape. Wash the bandages periodically in lukewarm water. Then drape them several times over a rod or line so that they dry without being stretched.

STEP THREE: Use leg vein–draining exercises to minimize congestion and to control leg weariness and cramps. Another way to break up the initial congestion of veins is with vein-draining exercises. They stop the vicious circle of congestion, veins dilated too far for their valves to work, more congestion, and so on. If veins have stretched so that valves don't close fully, pressure on the surface veins with support hose or bandages keeps blood from seesawing, enabling it to move on toward the heart. Often you won't realize how much congestion has affected you until you relieve it, whereupon night cramps and leg weariness disappear.

Whenever you need to stand still for long periods, take a break every hour or so. Remove your shoes. Lie on your back, and stretch your feet way up in the air, bracing your hips with both hands by planting your elbows on the surface on which you're lying. Keep your foot and calf muscles loose, and jiggle your feet for half a minute or more.

If you have only mild congestion in your leg veins, this exercise alone helps keep engorgement from progressing to the point where valves don't work. If your varicose veins in your lower leg exceed the diameter of a lead pencil, you need to combine support hose or bandaging with exercises.

Look at Bob W.'s case, for instance. As a forty-five-year-old barber, Bob stood up almost all through his workday. By quitting time, his legs felt so tired that he wondered whether they were going to just drop off. To make matters worse, he would lose an hour or so of sleep almost every night from leg cramps. His calf would knot up and hurt badly until he got up and walked around. Or he would get cramps in the arch of his foot.

When I looked at Bob's lower legs, engorged veins stood out like giant loops of blue spaghetti. I showed him how to collapse those surface vessels with elastic bandages, and explained leg vein–draining exercises.

A few months later, Bob's name was on the shop. Once he learned to keep those leg veins emptied out, he felt like a new man. His feet never got tired and the night cramps ceased. When the shop owner decided to retire, Bob took over the business. And he got the rest of the barbers doing the vein-draining exercise by setting up a spot for it in the back room. He found that the barbers all stayed a lot more cheerful and efficient when they could control vein congestion.

STEP FOUR: Consider surgery or injection treatment if leg cramps or great leg weariness caused by poor circulation persists. If cramps or great leg weariness persists, consider having a doctor inject or remove the varicose veins. Most of my patients who took that action said later that they didn't realize how much fatigue and discomfort the veins had been causing. They generally have remarked that if they had known how much better the operation would make them feel, they would have gone ahead with it much earlier.

CHAPTER
3

How to Keep Your Bones Strong and Fight Osteoporosis

When you think of old age, you probably think of bowed backs, pot bellies, and easily broken wrists or hips. But none of these problems comes from age itself; these problems come from *osteoporosis*. Osteoporosis, not age, weakens the fine slivers of bone inside the weight-bearing portions of your vertebrae. That lets the front portions of those structures crunch so that your back bows and your height decreases. These changes in your chest cage tip your ribs downward, which cuts into the available space for your internal organs and makes your abdomen bulge.

Osteoporosis, not age, leaches the strengthening calcium out of your wrist and hip bones. Even minor falls or impacts cause fractures that put you in a cast (or on the operating table).

If you stave off osteoporosis you'll stand tall and stay sturdy through all your years. Two out of every five women over forty have substantial bone thinning from osteoporosis. Almost the same proportion of men ultimately have this problem, but they get it somewhat later in life. Your *osteoporosis proneness index* tells how likely *you* are to have this disorder and how hard you should work at preventing it.

PRIME STRETCHER 1

Determine your osteoporosis proneness index.

Each of the available methods for staving off osteoporosis calls
for some expenditure of effort or change in your life-style. The
accompanying table shows you how to determine your *osteoporosis
proneness index* and will help you determine which measures,
if any, you need to take to prevent this condition.

Interpret your score according to this list:

- Over 100: Extreme risk. Should take all home measures
  described below, and consider hormone replacement (by
  prescription from your doctor).

- 80–100: Great risk. Follow all home measures described
  conscientiously.

- 50–80: Moderate risk. You can take some liberties, but
  should still follow my suggestions regarding diet and
  general exercise.

- Under 50: Minimal risk. Follow only suggestions that
  fit easily into your life-style.

---

*Mabel J. first came to me when she was forty-five. She
was very attractive—natural blonde hair, fine bones and
delicate skin. You could see even tiny vein branches on
the back of her hand, and her wrists and ankles were
very small.*

*I explained that unless she took countermeasures, these
characteristics made her likely to become bent and bowed
when she grew older. Mabel knew exactly what I was
talking about because she had seen it happen to her mother,
whom she said "just shriveled up before she was sixty."*

*Mabel and I went over the measures I'm going to explain
to you, and she stuck to them rigorously. She's sixty-eight
now, still straight-backed and dainty, standing as tall as*

OSTEOPOROSIS PRONENESS INDEX			
Trait	**Problem**	**Evaluation**	**Score**
Sex	Women have higher risk.	Females add 15.	
Age	Bone absorption increases with age.	Add 1 for each year above 40.	
Blonde?	Lighter complexion indicates more risk.	Blondes add 20, other whites 10, blacks 5.	
Slight?	Delicate build indicates risk. (Wrist circumference shows bone weight.)	Add 20 if delicate, 10 if medium, 0 if very rawboned.	
Skin quality	Thin transparent skin indicates high risk.	Add 20 if you can see small vein branches on the back of hands.	
Past menopause	Unreplaced lack of sex hormones cuts new bone formation.	Add 20 if past menopause (40 if ovaries removed early).*	
Diet	Lack of calcium and vitamins C and D hurts bone production.	Add 20 if you eat no dairy products, 10 if you don't eat them at least twice daily.	
Your personal osteoporosis proneness score =			

* Women can skip this item if hormone lack has always been replaced by prescribed estrogen-progesterone tablets or shots; score half if now replaced. Men suffer hormone lack only if testes have been removed or heavily irradiated (as for tumor). The "male menopause" doesn't count.

ever. (Her mother had lost 5 inches from her initially modest height.)

Mabel used every one of the following measures conscientiously.

PRIME STRETCHER 2

Make sure you have enough calcium in your diet.

Your body needs more calcium than any other mineral. Your nerves and muscles need a certain amount of calcium to function, and your system uses your bones as a reservoir for this crucial substance. If you don't absorb enough calcium from your food to make up for what your nerves and muscles lose, your body draws calcium out of your bones and this weakens them. Eating foods that contain calcium in a form your body can readily absorb keeps this from happening.

STEP ONE: Use lots of dairy products. You can get all the calcium you need from milk. Four glasses a day, whether skim, 1 percent, 2 percent or whole, provide an adequate amount of calcium to keep your bones sturdy. If you drink less milk,

- Eat yoghurt (equivalent ounce for ounce)
- Eat cottage cheese (twice the calcium per ounce)

STEP TWO: Use calcium tablets to fill out your calcium intake. Keep track of your total milk, yoghurt, and cottage cheese intake for one week. If your dairy product consumption falls short, get a supply of calcium lactate tablets (available without a prescription) or of Tums®. For each omitted glass of milk or equivalent, take two calcium lactate tablets or Tums® daily.

STEP THREE: Avoid calcium "blotters." Oxalic acid, contained in spinach, beet greens and rhubarb, keeps calcium from soaking into your system. So does phytic acid, contained in beans and other legumes and whole wheat, unless combined with yeast. (Beans can also be soaked in water for several hours, with the water then discarded, to remove phytic acid.) High-fiber cereals also blot up calcium and carry it through your bowel.

This doesn't mean that you can't eat these foods. Just don't count any calcium-containing food or drink that you take at the same meal with a "blotter" when you decide how many supplementary pills you need.

PRIME STRETCHER 3

Strengthen your bones through general exercise.

Getting enough calcium into your system is only half the battle. Getting your body to build bone substance out of that calcium is another matter. Exercise seems to be the key.

Mild but continuous exercise stirs your body to make stronger bones. Start with a 5-minute daily walk if you haven't been getting any exercise at all. Increase the duration and pace gradually until you are walking briskly for 20 minutes daily.

If walking doesn't appeal to you, what about swimming? You'll probably find a pool close by that you can use. Many schools open their pools to adults in the evening. Hospitals often have pools for patient rehabilitation, which they'll let you use at certain hours. You don't necessarily have to join an athletic club (or move South) just to swim.

PRIME STRETCHER 4

Use specific osteoporosis-fighting exercises.

Besides general body exercise, certain exercises help to prevent osteoporosis. If your osteoporosis risk is "great" or "extreme" according to the osteoporosis proneness index (or if you have any signs of the disease), you should do these special exercises once or twice a day:

1. Lie on your back. Grasp both knees and pull them toward your chest. Pull hard for 5 seconds.

2. While still on your back, put both legs out straight. Bring one knee up and pull it toward your chest with both hands, keeping the other leg entirely straight. Hold for 5 seconds. Repeat with the other leg.

3. Bend your knees until your feet are flat on the floor. Roll your hips forward as if doing a burlesque "bump," which should press the small of your back against the floor. Hold for 5 seconds.

4. Bend knees and fold your arms across your chest. Raise your head and shoulders a few inches off the floor. Hold for 3 seconds.

5. Keeping legs straight, arms flat at your sides, raise your head and shoulders. Hold 3 to 5 seconds.

6. Fold your arms in front of your chest and bring your bent knees up close to them. Slowly straighten your legs, keeping your heels at the same height from the floor. Slowly return to starting position.

7. Bend your knees with feet flat on floor. Fold your hands behind your head. Press both elbows against the floor for 5 seconds.

8. Tuck your chin down against your chest. Squeeze your shoulder blades together strongly for 5 seconds.

9. Roll over onto your stomach with a pillow underneath your chest. Keep your chin tucked down against your chest. Squeeze shoulder blades together firmly for 5 seconds.

These movements strengthen the muscles that support your spine. As your muscles build up, you can do each exercise two, three, or four times each session.

PRIME STRETCHER 5

Retain more of the calcium in your body.

You can also take steps to cut down the amount of calcium that passes out of your system.

STEP ONE: Get enough vitamin D, but be sure to avoid excess. To control osteoporosis you need 400 milligrams (mg.) of vitamin D a day, which you will almost certainly get from enriched milk, butter, or margarine. However, daily intake over 1,000 mg. actually harms calcium absorption, so you should check the labels on any vitamin preparations (or calcium-vitamin combinations) you use to be sure you don't add more than 600 mg. to that in natural food sources.

The next two measures are tougher. But if you have great or extreme osteoporosis risk, they're definitely worth the sacrifice.

STEP TWO: Give up or cut way down on the foods and beverages that cause calcium to pass out of your body through your urine. These include excess red meat, sugar, salt, chocolate, coffee, soft drinks, and processed meats.

STEP THREE: Stop smoking if you haven't already done so (see page 294 for help). Nicotine makes calcium pour through your system into your urine, which you just can't afford if you're fighting a high osteoporosis risk.

PRIME STRETCHER 6

Start a bone-strengthening program if you already have osteoporosis.

It's never too late to start your bone-strengthening program. You can take all the measures I've advised after osteoporosis starts. You can also do a lot for yourself if a vertebra begins to collapse.

STEP ONE: Recognize and take countermeasures if vertebrae compress. Vertebral fractures usually happen while you are lifting something or when you get a sudden upward jar or jolt (as from a fall). You get sudden pain at one level of your backbone, usually between your shoulder blades.

You'll probably be able to feel or see an unevenness in the spacing or prominence of your backbone's knobs. This will tell you for sure which vertebra has collapsed and make it easier for you to follow this approach:

1. Go to bed. Be sure your sleep surface is very firm. If it isn't, get a cotton mattress and a bed board to put on top.

2. Partly fill a sandwich-size Ziploc® bag with sand, exhausting the air before you seal it. Place it inside a larger bag (as a precaution against leaks). Put this under the sore vertebra, which makes your body weight tend to pull the compressed area apart. This will relieve pain and reduce later deformity.

3. Stay in bed for a week or ten days, by which time you should be able to stand up for a few minutes at a time. Increase your "up" time, resting for a few minutes whenever the soreness increases, until healing is complete.

4. While in bed, do leg vein–draining exercises every hour. Raise your feet as far as possible. With your ankle muscles loose, jiggle your feet rapidly for 1 minute.

5. Remain alert for leg vein clots, which are the main hazard of bed rest. Although leg vein–draining exercises usually prevent this condition, check every day (even after you are getting up some) for swelling of one or both ankles or tenderness in one or both calves. If either occurs, see your doctor right away.

Bed rest keeps pain to a minimum. It also may help to keep the damaged vertebra from collapsing further, perhaps to the point where nerve pressure occurs.

STEP TWO: Use an abdominal binder to lessen back discomfort.
When you first get up, you may find that an abdominal binder
helps prolong the interval before pain makes you go back to
bed. You can get a factory-made Velcro® binder at your drugstore
or hospital supply store. Or you can cut and hem a piece of
bleached muslin wide enough to cover your entire abdomen
and long enough to overlap about 8 inches in the front. Use
six or eight large safety pins to hold the latter snug.

To put the binder on, stand up and take a deep breath.
Draw in your abdomen. Pull the binder tight while your stomach
is flat and fasten it with the Velcro® or the pins. Wear it under
your clothes until bedtime.

As soon as you can do so comfortably, start the spine-
supporting muscle strengthening exercises described earlier.
These strengthen muscles that brace the injured area. They help
both in easing the soreness and in minimizing deformity.

---

*Harriet S. was only 46, but she already had osteoporosis.
One day while doing her weekly wash, she lifted a basket
of wet clothes. Pain hit suddenly between her shoulder
blades. It felt as if someone had shot her with an arrow.
She put down the basket and laid on the sofa for a while.
That helped, but her back still hurt almost all the time.
And the pain would shoot right through her when she
coughed or sneezed.*

*Harriet's back pain came from a collapsed vertebra. She
spent the next week in bed; then she gradually mobilized
herself over the following two weeks. She had to lie down
for 15 minutes every 2 or 3 hours for about two months
before the pain left.*

*Harriet started the preventive program I've just explained.
I was afraid she might have one or two more collapsed
vertebrae before the program took hold, but luckily she
hasn't had any further trouble.*

PRIME STRETCHER 7

*Intensify your osteoporosis program after
any wrist or hip fracture.*

Over the years, I've seen dozens of patients who had
this succession of events:

1. A fractured wrist or hip, with X rays showing apparently
   normal bone density (no osteoporosis diagnosed, at
   least)

2. Normal healing of said fracture

3. Years later, a crunched vertebra, at which time studies
   showed distinct osteoporosis

So I now make these recommendations to every patient
with a wrist or hip fracture:

- Even if you were run over by a truck or otherwise
  injured in a way that makes the fracture seem to have
  purely external causes, consider it evidence of weakened
  bone structure.

- Go back to the osteoporosis proneness index table and
  add 40 points to your previous score.

- Follow the more intensive routine your new score suggests.

- *Stick with that routine!* It's hard to keep at it year after
  year when you have no complaints. But you're almost
  sure to have another fracture (wrist, hip, or crunched
  vertebra) within ten years if you don't.

CHAPTER 4

Sex for Seniors: A Key to Staying Younger Longer

Many people talk as if for seniors, sex is only a memory. They tell "old man" jokes and label marriage between people in their sixties (or even fifties) as "companionate." Whether they realize it or not, they continually support the myth that sex is the exclusive province of the young.

First, this notion is blatantly untrue. Healthy men and women can remain sexually active into their seventies and eighties.

Second, this myth can undermine the confidence you need to enjoy life to its fullest, and it can actually rob you of your sexual capacities.

PRIME STRETCHER 1

Don't let false myths upset you, inhibit you, or rob you of potency.

When I gave a sex education class to a group of high school seniors, the only thing I said which shocked them was: "Of course, your parents still have sexual intercourse. In fact, it's so much more convenient for them that they probably have it a lot more often than you do."

Being staunchly imbued with the American myth that sex belongs strictly to youth, the students' mouths literally dropped open. I don't know what they would have done if I had mentioned grandparents too!

Think about movies that have portrayed older women as sexually active. From Mrs. Robinson in *The Graduate* to Ava Gardner with her "beach boys" in *Night of the Iguana*, they've all been shown as somehow immoral.

And when a younger man goes around with an older woman, what do some people say? "He's after her money" is a lot more common than "Really attractive, isn't she?" But she quite probably *is* attractive! And there's nothing wrong or abnormal about her still being interested and involved.

If you're a woman, the menopause doesn't cut down either your attractiveness or your sex urge. Actually, once you don't have to worry about pregnancy, you may find that your interest increases, and your greater responsiveness increases your appeal! If you find yourself in this position, don't let our society's false myths make you feel guilty. Don't let them burden your sex life with furtiveness or concealment.

Of course, you might not feel this way at all. Sex urge or interest varies widely at any age; if you honestly don't feel any need or desire, that's perfectly normal, too. But let *your own* feelings, not the false American mythology, govern. Whether you're interested and active or not, don't think less of yourself or feel guilty.

If you're a man, and if you've let any of this "sex is the property of youth" malarkey soak in, your first step toward maintaining your sex life is to root it out. You need to realize that occasional inability to get or sustain an erection doesn't mean that you're "over the hill." That's how the false rumor of the "male menopause" takes its toll. Almost every man has occasional total or partial impotence. You can usually trace these episodes to one of the problems we'll soon discuss. But if you're imbued with the idea of the "male menopause," you might not even try to be sexually active! You just think: "That's it! I've lost my powers." Then lack of confidence and anxiety make you fail the next time, too. And pretty soon the "male menopause" prophecy will have made itself come true and robbed you of your potency!

This never has to happen. If occasionally you can't get a firm and lasting erection, just shrug and say to yourself: "I'll be all right next time." And if you *aren't* all right and the problem becomes frequent or constant, *don't* just shrug: use the next few pages to identify and conquer the source of your impotence, which is *never* just age!

PRIME STRETCHER 2

If impaired potency is a problem, nocturnal erections help you to discover the cause.

Before you can do anything about impotence, you need to know whether it comes from a *physical* or a *nonphysical* condition. Any physical cause makes *all* erections impossible, including nocturnal erections or so-called "bladder erections" (because when you wake up with one you usually need to void before it subsides).

STEP ONE: Check the presence or absence of nocturnal erections to sort out physical from emotional or relationship-related impotence. If you generally woke up during the night with a bladder erection before you became impotent, you can be absolutely sure that

- If bladder erections have disappeared, the cause of your impotence is *physical.*

- If bladder erections occur even occasionally, the physical equipment works, and your problem lies in the *emotional* or *relationship* area.

Very complex and expensive procedures done in sleep disorder centers have proved that a man always gets at least a partial erection if he sleeps soundly enough to reach plane III, the sleep phase during which you dream and your eyes move underneath your eyelids. However, you may not wake up when this occurs, so you might not be aware of it. If you don't know whether or not you have nocturnal erections, here's how to check.

STEP TWO: Use this home technique to check for nocturnal erections. If nocturnal erections don't awaken you enough to make you aware of them, you can check for their occurrence with this simple home technique:

1. Cut a 2-inch by 5-inch piece out of an old handkerchief or shirt tail.

2. Obtain some draftsman's tape or masking tape. These tapes are just sticky enough to hold things in place if there's no strain on the joint, but will release if under stress.

3. Do not drink alcohol or take sleeping pills on the night of the test. (These interfere with plane III sleep.)

4. At bedtime, wrap the cloth snugly but not tightly around the base of your penis. Use 3 inches of the draftsman's or masking tape to hold the overlapping end of the cloth to the underlying layer. Do not let the tape overlap onto the skin.

5. Get a good night's sleep, without disturbing the cloth. If you do not sleep well, repeat for several nights until you do.

6. If the cloth remains in place undisturbed after a good night's sleep, your impotence almost certainly has a physical cause.

STEP THREE: If prior steps aren't conclusive, a doctor can arrange for a definitive test in a sleep disorder center. Any doctor (not necessarily a specialist) can arrange for a test that uses brain waves to show what sleep plane you have reached and wrap a pressure-sensitive cuff around the penis to check for erection. This test is done in a sleep disorder center because of the equipment needed, even though your problem has nothing to do with sleep. The test is expensive but 100 percent certain and is certainly worthwhile if you need it to sort out the nature of a problem with potency.

PRIME STRETCHER 3

*Cure some forms of physically caused
impotence with vitamins.*

Certain nerves signal your blood vessels to trap blood in the penis and give you an erection. These nerves can use only simple sugars (normally glucose) as fuel. The conditions we're about to discuss block your nerve cells from using glucose. This is a frequent cause of impotence. But large amounts of vitamin B make alternate metabolic paths available. This can let those crucial nerves function again.

If you lose potency because of any of the conditions we're going to discuss next (all of which impair normal use of glucose in your nerve cells and disturb your potency), here's what you should do:

1. Select a vitamin supplement that contains vitamin B only. Don't use one-a-day complete vitamin-mineral formulas. To get the amount of B you need to correct impotence from such capsules would involve harmful overdose of A and D.

2. Be sure the formula has all B vitamins in proper proportion. Large amounts of one B vitamin encourage your body to use sugars in a way that increases demand for other B's. Too much B_1 without extra B_2 can give you the same complaints you would get from a total lack of B_2. Some inexpensive products (and some "megavitamins" at health food stores) have a lot of the inexpensive B_1 without matching amounts of the more expensive B_2. A balanced formula should come close to having multiples of the minimum daily requirement (MDR) amounts shown in the box. In particular, the B_2 should be at least as much as the B_1.

3. Take enough of this balanced formula to give you at least 30 mg. of B_1 (thiamine) every day. (Overdose of straight B complex won't hurt.)

MDRs of Vitamin B Complex

B_1	Thiamine	1.5 mg.
B_2	Rioflavin	1.7 mg.
	Niacinamide	20.0 mg.
B_6	Pyridoxine	2.0 mg.
B_{12}	Cyanocobalamin	6.0 mcg.

STEP ONE: Use vitamins to cure impotence from past privation.

Reverend Jerry B.'s case showed me just how long the metabolic scars of privation could last. Rev. Jerry had survived the Bataan death march and years in a Japanese prison camp. He had even given part of his meager food rations to soldiers he felt were more in need (most of whom died anyway). When finally freed, his 6'2" body weighed 102 pounds. When I saw him ten years later, he weighed 185. But even though he had a normal diet and life-style since his captivity, he had never been able to get an erection.

Rev. Jerry's body's way of burning glucose had been permanently harmed by the period of deprival. A normal body's main way of burning sugars needs only modest amounts of vitamin B. It burns sugars in a way that uses vitamins only temporarily and completely regenerates them. But starvation had destroyed some of the enzymes Rev. Jerry needed to burn sugars in that way. His body had fallen back on an alternate mechanism that needs large amounts of B_1 and B_2 because it uses these substances up instead of regenerating them. Without large amounts of vitamins B_1 and B_2, certain crucial nerves just couldn't function.

> *After two weeks of high vitamin B intake, Rev. Jerry had normal erections. He has no further problems, as long as he keeps up the vitamins.*

Chances are you didn't survive a death march or years in a prison camp. But you may well have survived a period of malnutrition.

One study of black males reared in the South during the 1950s and 60s showed 40 percent impotence. The author was a psychiatrist who blamed "performance anxiety from unrealistic expectations" (a distinctly racist pronouncement which I apologize for having to quote). But virtually all the black men whom I have treated for impotence and who were reared during that era of economic inequity had suffered periods of privation. Most were cured by vitamins.

Even well-to-do people can go through periods of malnutrition—for example, teenage rebellion against parental rules, fad diets, and so on. A nutritionist studied diets of high school students in the wealthy suburb of Edina, Minnesota, and found that almost half had inadequate diets. Some of the deficiencies were mild, but a few were severe enough to make lifelong enzyme damage seem probable.

If you have ever lived alone, you may not have eaten nutritiously. The only patient I have ever seen with full blown beriberi, the disease caused by total lack of vitamin B_1, was a well-to-do widower who solved the "cooking problem" by eating nothing but canned baked beans three meals a day.

Even if you have eaten a well-balanced diet for many years, past privation can still be a factor in impotence. If so, you may have had occasional or frequent poor quality erections—ones barely sufficient to permit intercourse. This makes it almost certain that your impotence is nutritional. Or you might not have any trouble at all for years until other erection-undermining factors, including emotional ones, add to the residuals of privation. Whether nutritional factors are the whole cause or only part of the cause of impotence, vitamins will help.

STEP TWO: Use vitamins to control alcohol-related impotence.
Alcohol may spur the urge toward sex, but it often takes away
the power to indulge in it. Alcohol works by affecting the
way your brain cells use glucose, so a period of alcoholic excess
can permanently damage your nerve cell metabolism, just as
starvation or deprivation can. Even moderate amounts of alcohol,
used continually over a period of years, can cause lasting impotence, especially if your family history includes the other
great sugar-use abnormality, diabetes.

If you're a "social drinker" and become impotent, try quitting alcohol for a few weeks, and take vitamin B. The vitamins
alone won't do the trick if you keep drinking, and quitting
usually won't restore potency promptly without vitamins. Even
if you give up alcohol for years, impotence may persist if you
drank heavily enough to damage your system. If impotence
began while you were drinking, try vitamins for at least a
month. Response often takes considerable time, but often ultimately occurs.

STEP THREE: Use vitamins to combat impotence from diabetes.
Diabetes profoundly affects your body's way of burning glucose,
so it often causes impotence.

Providing alternate channels of glucose use by the nervous
system through large doses of vitamins often helps. But you
need full doses for a long time—sometimes two or three months
for full effect.

————————————————————

*Mike S. had done a good job of controlling his diabetes.
He kept every blood sugar reading right on the mark,
but still had totally lost potency. There was no way
to improve Mike's way of managing his disease. I suggested that high doses of vitamin B might give his
body an alternate way of using sugars and restore his
potency.*

*After a month he reported improvement—"enough to get
in, but still not really solid." In three months he reported*

*"good, firm erections," which have been available to him
ever since, so long as he continues the vitamins.*

If you have any evidence of present or impending diabetes,[1]
getting it under careful control will help you to "stretch your
prime" in many ways, including maintained potency. You may
still need vitamins to help potency, and you may need to take
them for two or three months before you know whether they're
going to help.

PRIME STRETCHER 4

*Relieve toxic impotence by changing habits
or medications.*

If impotence kills all your erections, including nocturnal erections,
and none of the causes we've discussed seems to fit, chances
are it's a side effect of a medication. Almost any substance
that can affect either blood vessels (which make the penis erect
by filling it with blood under high pressure) or nerves (which
tell the blood vessels what to do) can make you impotent. All
these common medications can sometimes interfere with one
or the other part of the mechanism:

- Blood pressure pills
- Heart rhythm regulators
- Anticonvulsants
- Stomach acid inhibitors (Tagomet®)
- Antispasmodics containing atropine or hyoscine
- Tranquilizers
- Sedatives

---

[1] Tests showing what happens to your blood sugar after a high-carbohydrate meal
may show a tendency toward diabetes several years before you have full-fledged
diabetes with sugar in your urine or high blood sugar readings. Mild control measures
at that stage may keep the disease at bay for many extra years.

- Motion sickness drugs
- Antinauseants
- Hemorrhoid or fissure suppositories
- Eye drops

"Maybe it's all over for me," Allen P. said to me. "But fifty-two seems awful young to lose out on sex."

Allen never had any trouble whatever with his erections until about six weeks before that visit. Then they became less and less firm. At first, he could still complete the sex act. But by the time he came to my office, his impotence had become complete. Even nocturnal erections had ceased entirely.

In Allen's case, one of the most common physical causes seemed likely: his blood pressure pills. Even though he had taken the same medication for years without trouble, I switched him to a different type. Inside of a week, his erections were back to their former strength.

You'll usually need a doctor's help to replace offending medications. But most of them *can* be replaced. If you just assume that you've hit the "male menopause," both you and your partner can lose out on years of an enjoyable sex life.

PRIME STRETCHER 5

Get help from a urologist if home measures fail.

If impotence has wiped out nocturnal erections and none of the remedies just suggested fit your case, a urologist can often help.

Prostate infection, which very commonly causes impotence, usually responds to prescribed antibiotics. Even if a smoldering infection persists, a urologist can draw out congestion from the gland periodically, which often restores potency.

As a last resort, a urologist can surgically implant a device that will let you have intercourse. Modern implants can be pumped up and deflated, so they don't interfere with comfort when not in use. Failure to get a natural erection does not interfere with sensation, so you can enjoy sex as much as usual.

PRIME STRETCHER 6

Restore potency by getting rid of depression.

If your impotence is accompanied by two or more of these signs, chances are you have depression caused by altered brain chemistry:

- Blue moods, especially in the morning

- Loss of interest in things you've previously enjoyed

- Crying, or feeling as if you ought to cry, especially when alone

- Awakening at 2 or 3 A.M. and not being able to get back to sleep

- Loss of appetite and weight

- Constipation

You can't just "buck up" or change the things that seem to be getting you down with this disorder. You need antidepressant medications.

The appropriate medicines can't be bought without a prescription, so you'll have to see a doctor. These medications usually work, but only after two or three weeks—sometimes even longer. Don't get discouraged if considerable time goes by before you see results.

PRIME STRETCHER 7

Combat performance anxiety by setting no goals, by focusing primarily on pleasurable sensations, and by getting your partner to be totally undemanding.

One marriage counselor with whom I have worked speaks disparagingly of "Pleasers." He cures some men of impotence by getting them to focus entirely on their own pleasure, with total disregard for their partner's.

That's going too far, in my opinion. But trying to "shoot par" can involve enough anxiety to kill potency, whether you set that "par" for yourself with unrealistic expectations (like mutual orgasm) or your partner sets them for you with unrealistic demands or expressed dissatisfactions.

Three measures will help restore potency impaired in this way:

1. Just let sex happen. Don't set goals for frequency, duration, or particularly for elicited response.

2. Focus on your own feelings sufficiently to both enjoy them and to let your partner know (by word or gesture) what she can do to improve your pleasure.

3. Insist that your partner demand nothing that doesn't occur naturally through interaction.

The perfect partner for helping you overcome impotence from performance anxiety takes all pressure off by indicating satisfaction no matter what, makes herself constantly available, and gives you support and approval instead of belittlement and demands. That's asking a lot. But your partner has a lot to gain by improving your performance. If you can convince her that she will also get more enjoyment during sex if she cooperates, perhaps she'll be willing.

PRIME STRETCHER 8

Develop outlets for accumulated anger, which commonly causes either frigidity or impotence.

If (as a man) you get an erection during sex play or anticipation, but lose it when you try to have intercourse, or (as a woman) you find yourself unable to respond sexually, *accumulated anger* is usually the cause.

Whenever someone does something that displeases you, you react emotionally. Since "loss of self-control" (which includes getting angry) is one of the few taboos in our society, most of us don't call this particular spade a spade. We "resent" our partner's sloppiness around the house. We "get exasperated" at tracked-in dirt. We "feel disappointed in" spouses who stay in bed instead of getting up to fix breakfast.

All the phrases I've put in quotation marks really mean anger.

Both frigidity and impotence often come from anger, but not from raging anger at some major affront. It is usually caused by accumulated, smoldering anger from a dozen trivial events—matters nowhere nearly as important to either of you as your relationship.

So what can you do about it?

1. Air your gripes. Anything that annoys you deserves attention *now*. Otherwise, you'll smolder along and ultimately blow up over something even more inconsequential.

2. Talk about your feelings, not the other person's acts. You *help* your relationship when you say: "It upset me when you more or less called me a souse by telling Jim not to give me another drink." You *hurt* your relationship when you say: "What's the matter with you? Pushing me around like that? Might as well have called me an alcoholic!" And believe it or not, you hurt your relationship *even more* if you don't say anything at all!

That anger will keep eating at you, and come out in ways which don't tell your partner what he or she needs to do to keep you happy—often by a later episode of unresponsiveness or impotence.

3. Develop other outlets for residual anger, like sports: hitting, stabbing, or shooting something can be an outlet for feelings you haven't recognized or acknowledged.

Harvey S. complained of impotence, but he still got nocturnal erections almost every night. At age fifty-three, he had been "happily married" for over twenty years. But for the past six months, he had been having more and more trouble with his sex life. He would get a partial or full erection during sex play, but then lose it when he tried to have intercourse. I could tell right away that he didn't have anything wrong physically. If you can get an erection any time, you can get one and hold it for sex.

Harvey had no signs of depression, so it seemed worthwhile to take another look at his "happy" marriage. I suggested that the three of us—Harvey, his wife Maude and I—get together once.

Actually, it took more than once. Maude came into the sessions with a chip on her shoulder, thinking I was blaming her for everything. When we worked that through, she came up with a whole list of complaints about Harvey, ranging from his getting high and flirting with lady friends to coming in from the yard with muddy shoes. Actually, what she had done to annoy Harvey turned out to be mostly after-effects of his own behavior—rejecting sexual advances while smoldering with anger about the flirting, calling him a "filthy slob" for tracking in dirt.

We went through a considerable procedure to heal these wounds. Both Harvey and Maude drew up lists of changes they would like to see the other make. They talked about what approaches might work out; then they wrote up a little "contract." Maude agreed to be "available" and Harvey to be considerate in a dozen or so specific ways.

That formal agreement helped them give each other a chance. And they found that each one really did still mean a lot to the other. All they really needed was a way of getting trivial gripes on the table. Once they could see what they were doing to irritate each other, and how unimportant most of the issues were (except for the resentment they stirred), their real liking for one another took hold.

"We're doing fine together now," Harvey told me at our last visit. "And we've got our 'contract' down to two words. 'Don't smolder'—anything gripes either of us, he or she decides 'What the hell, I'll go along with that for the sake of the relationship' or we get it on the table right away. No more tit-for-tat that builds and builds."

"And no more trouble with erections?"

"No indeed!"

PRIME STRETCHER 9

Stave off the female menopause.

No one can deny that *women* have a menopause. That event has deep significance, but you don't have to let it disturb either your physical health, your emotions, or your sex life.

Countless studies have proven that *sexual activity makes your ovaries continue to produce its hormones.* One such study [2] compared nuns with prostitutes. The average nun had her menopause in her thirties, the average prostitute in her fifties. That's quite a difference! It means that you can stave off the menopause by remaining sexually active.

---

[2] Conducted in Italy, where prostitution was legal at the time.

- If you have intercourse at least weekly, you're keeping your ovaries fully active.

- Self-stimulation to orgasm has the same hormone-producing effect.

PRIME STRETCHER 10

Manage the physical complaints of menopause.

Most people think that the menopause inevitably means hot flashes, headaches, and uncomfortable skin sensations. Actually, you have better than a 50–50 chance of escaping these problems, especially if you stay sexually active. (The nuns in the study cited often had hot flashes, the prostitutes almost never.)

If these complaints do prove aggravating, take these steps:

1. Every orgasm gets your ovaries to make the hormones you need to combat menopausal symptoms, so remain sexually active. The measures I suggested for staving off the menopause also help to relieve symptoms that accompany it.

2. Menopausal headaches respond better to aspirin, Tylenol®, or ibuprofen if you take a cup or two of strong coffee at the same time.

3. For hot flashes, dress in removable layers. Carry a moist handkerchief in a plastic bag wherever you go. Apply a cold cloth to the back of your neck or to your forehead when the flash occurs.

4. Don't be afraid to take medically prescribed hormones if you need them for relief. Such hormones actually prolong your life[3] as well as relieve your symptoms.

---

[3] Hormones cut your risk of heart disease and of osteoporosis-related wrist, hip, and spine fractures. This adds almost twice as much life expectancy as you lose through increased uterine and breast cancer.

PRIME STRETCHER 11

Avoid "menopause baby" pregnancies.

Age alone is no guide to the end of fertility, nor is the end of menstruation an immediate sign. Periods always become irregular before ovarian activity ends completely, so you need to continue using contraceptives during the menopausal years. Here's how to manage it:

1. Continue to use contraceptives for two full years after your last period. Every year thousands of women get pregnant months after they thought they were "finished with all that." An unwanted pregnancy after your "first family" graduates can seem disastrous. In some abortion clinics, such cases outnumber the unmarried teenagers two to one.

2. Give up the pill. The cycle it imposes continues to cause monthly bleeding even if your natural fertility has ceased. You have to shift to another birth control method before you can tell when you can stop using contraceptives.

3. Try foam. If you can tolerate an interruption in preliminary play, insert two plungers-full, or use it in anticipation. Although the directions say to use foam "immediately before intercourse," a few minutes make no difference. You can get ready at bedtime or whenever you think you might need contraception. (You do need to use a fresh dose for "repeats," though, even if they occur quite promptly. Secretions from the first episode dilute the materials too much to let you count on them again.)

4. If you can't (or don't like to) use foam, try spermicidal suppositories or creams. The extra lubrication that makes these products unsuitable for young women often proves to be an advantage after the menopause, when natural lubrication lessens.

5. You may be able to use a cervical cap. When menstrual flow doesn't occur to displace it, this creates a lasting barrier to penetrating sperm. You'll need to get this fitted by a doctor.

6. As a last resort, consider surgical interruption of your Fallopian tubes. A gynecologist can do this using an instrument, without an operation. The procedure involves virtually no disability or pain. The expense may or may not be covered by your insurance, which you'll want to find out before making your first visit to the doctor.

7. You'll notice that I haven't mentioned the diaphragm. Changes in vaginal contour during intercourse keep even the best-fitted diaphragm from acting as a barrier to penetrating sperm. The number of failures (about one for each ten years of childbearing age) is exactly the same as for spermicidal jelly alone. But the diaphragm does keep spermicidal jelly in place until intercourse. This means that you can insert it well in advance whenever you think you might need protection. Balance that factor against the diaphragm-caused impaired sensation for you and your partner, and then decide whether a diaphragm is right for you.

8. Don't use an intrauterine device (IUD). These frequently cause bleeding, which creates two problems: first, you need extensive tests to be sure you don't have a tumor, and, second, you can't tell whether the bleeding shows continued ovarian activity, requiring another two years of contraception.

9. Consider these points in making your final choice:

   • Only surgery is 100 percent effective.

   • Foam comes next if used *every time*.[4]

   • Spermicidal suppositories or jellies, with or without a diaphragm, are the third most efficient.

---

[4] This statement is based on "method failures"—pregnancies despite uniform use. "Total failures," which include pregnancies due to failing to use the procedure, are almost the same for the diaphragm with spermicide.

- Creams, jellies, and suppositories give lubrication as well as contraception, which may be an advantage if your vaginal glands have become less active.

PRIME STRETCHER 12

Keep your vagina strong and moist.

After the menopause, your vaginal walls become thinner and the glands that make natural lubricant function less actively. You can keep these changes from affecting your sex life in several ways:

- An active sex life itself reduces vaginal changes. If you have no partner and you have no objections on moral grounds, self-stimulation accomplishes this goal.

- Strengthen the surrounding muscles with Kegel's exercises. You may have done these exercises to restore pelvic muscle strength after having a baby. Your goal is to contract the muscles of the pelvic floor for 3 to 5 seconds, relax for a few seconds, contract again, and so on. Practice contracting these muscles by cutting off the flow of urine several times during a voiding. You can also pretend you are picking up marbles with your vagina, or try to pull your anal opening up inside your body. Use whichever self-command tightens the muscles best. Do this twenty to thirty times at a session, and try to get in a hundred contractions a day. It sounds like a lot, but you can do this exercise while you're talking on the phone, driving your car, or working at your desk, so it really doesn't take up any time.

- Use a glycerine-based lubricant if needed. K-Y Jelly®, obtainable in any drugstore, lubricates well but has a clinical scent. More aesthetically pleasing lubricants can be obtained from sex-supply stores or catalogs. Don't use petroleum jellies (like Vaseline®)—vaginal infections sometimes follow their use.

PRIME STRETCHER 13

Accommodate the age-sensitized clitoris.

The tissue thinning that occurs after the menopause increases the exposure of your clitoris (the sensitive erectile nub at the front of your vagina's inner lips). The increased sensitivity that results calls for some adjustments in your sexual practices.

- Lubricate the clitoral area with K-Y® or other glycerine-based jelly when you anticipate intercourse.
- Speak up. Caresses and sex positions that were pleasant at one phase of your sex life may be uncomfortable or downright painful with greater clitoral exposure. Unless you explain this to your partner, he'll never know.

PRIME STRETCHER 14

Avoid postmenopausal "honeymoon cystitis."

As the years go by, your bladder becomes less insulated from your vagina. The vaginal wall becomes thinner when the production of ovarian hormones decreases. Intervening fibrous tissues, especially if stretched by childbirth, diminish and weaken. The tube leading from the bladder to the exterior becomes wider and more lax.

These changes make the thrust of the penis more likely to cause bladder irritation. They also make it easier for sexual activity to move germs up the urethra into the bladder and cause infection. To avoid these problems, take these steps:

1. Drink lots of water before and after sex. Copious flow of fluid washes away germs.
2. Empty your bladder shortly after intercourse. This will wash away germs that have been pushed part way up the urinary passage.
3. If bladder irritation occurs, try flooding your system with water. Increasing urinary volume sometimes

washes away irritants and gives relief. But if irritation continues, or if it is accompanied by fever, see your doctor.

PRIME STRETCHER 15

Don't let physical disabilities stop you.

You don't need to give up sex if either you or your partner develops physical disabilities.

Gentle sex play still conveys both affection and pleasure. If either you or your partner just can't manage anything more, don't be afraid that a few caresses will "start something you can't finish." Mature people can settle for what's available, and a little love is better than none.

Mutual play to climax calls for much less exertion and potential discomfort than intercourse. After a heart attack, for instance, you (or your partner) can enjoy play-induced orgasms two weeks after you get home from the hospital. It is wise to wait at least six weeks before having intercourse. If severe arthritis, stroke, or other disability makes intercourse impossible, play to climax remains as a sound means of making love.

Intercourse with both partners lying on their sides and the husband approaching from the rear puts less strain on both partners' hearts and bodies. You can enjoy love-making in this way with many conditions that would trouble you in other postures.

PRIME STRETCHER 16

Overcome the effects of breast or uterine surgery.

If you need to have surgery performed on your breasts or female organs, these steps should help:

- After breast surgery, explore other erogenous zones during sex play. Gentle stimulation of the earlobes and ear openings or the conjunctiva (through the eyelids) builds sexual excitement as thoroughly as stimulation of the nipples.

- Realize that your appeal to your partner remains unimpaired. Most of the couples I have followed through breast surgery have been drawn closer by having gone through an ordeal together. None have been pulled apart.

- Understand that removal of your uterus has no effect whatever on your sexual appeal or your sex life.

- Ovarian cysts do *not* come from venereal disease. (Two of my patients had previously broken off important relationships because of this misconception.)

CHAPTER
5

Overcome Urinary Difficulties with Self-help Techniques

Do you take automatic urinary control and easy, comfortable passing of urine for granted? As the years go by, these functions may not be so easy! Several of the most common plagues of advancing years affect elimination, including

- Stress incontinence, which soils undergarments when a cough, sneeze, or sometimes even a hearty laugh sends a wave of pressure to your bladder. A great many women, especially mothers of two or more children, and a few men suffer from this condition.

- Incontinence following prostate surgery or nervous system injury or disorder.

- Bladder infection or irritation.

- Bulging of the bladder or rectum into the vagina, causing cystocele or rectocele.

- Prostate problems.

PRIME STRETCHER 1

Improve urinary control with a special exercise.

Your urine flows to the surface through a narrow tube called the urethra. Near that tube's junction with your bladder, a ring of special muscle surrounds it. This is one of the few muscles in your body that you control by *relaxing* instead of *contracting* it. As long as you don't think about it, this ring of muscle stays snug and cuts off the flow of urine. When you "let go" on purpose, the muscle relaxes and allows urine to pass.

This means that you have to learn deliberately to contract the cut-off-the-stream muscle before you can strengthen it. Several circumstances make that process worthwhile.

If you're a woman, especially if you have borne several children, loss of a few drops of urine when you cough or sneeze becomes quite likely after age forty. If you're a man, incontinence occurs quite commonly after surgery on your prostate. It's a lot easier to learn to contract the appropriate muscles while you're voiding normally and can tell what cuts off the stream than when an operation has interrupted your patterns.

STEP ONE: Learn to contract the cut-off-the-stream muscle, when the only conscious control you have previously had relaxes it. You'll find it almost impossible to single out one muscle in your pelvic floor and contract it. The same nerve bundles that control the muscles that cut off the urinary stream also govern the other muscles of the pelvic floor, and all muscles supplied by one nerve generally contract at once.

Different people find different self-commands effective in making the pelvic floor muscles contract. Try each of these:

1. Cut off the flow of urine several times during a voiding.

2. Pretend you are picking up marbles with your vagina.

3. Try to pull your anal opening up inside your body.

STEP TWO: Use the most effective command to strengthen your pelvic floor muscles. You will feel the muscles firm up to a different extent with each of these commands. Use whichever one tightens the muscles best. Keep the muscles tight for 5 seconds, relax briefly, then repeat. Do this twenty times at a session, and try to get in a hundred contractions a day. It sounds like a lot, but you can do this exercise while you're talking on the phone, driving your car, or working at your desk. It really doesn't take up any time, and after a while requires almost no concentration.

STEP THREE: After thorough control has been established, keep at least one session of twenty contractions in your weekly routines. The one trouble with using exercises to solve a health problem is that you tend to quit when the problem disappears. In this case, you don't need to work as hard maintaining muscle strength as you worked building it. Just pick one thing you do every week, like read the Sunday paper, and do your pelvic floor exercises simultaneously.

STEP FOUR: If stress incontinence persists, consider surgical relief. The idea of having an operation in this area is quite frightening, but the procedure doctors use to correct this problem is quite safe and involves very little discomfort. If incontinence is sufficient to be a real embarrassment, it's a shame to put up with it when a relatively minor operation should give relief.

PRIME STRETCHER 2

Don't let incontinence isolate or sideline you.

If you let it, the possible embarrassment of even mild incontinence can greatly harm your life-style. I have seen patients who let the prospect of slight urine leakage make them virtual recluses. Yet chances are no one will ever know about mild to moderate incontinence unless you tell them about it.

You can handle mild incontinence in the same way whether you're a woman or a man.

STEP ONE: Anoint the area. Before using a pad or other means to catch stray urine, you should use a protective ointment on any tissue that will be in contact with the wet pad. Diaprene®, found with baby products at your drugstore, works very well. If the tissue is already scalded by urinary irritants, use zinc oxide ointment until the irritation subsides. You'll find that the ointments spread much thinner if you let a few dabs warm up on your skin for a minute or two before rubbing them around.

STEP TWO: Use just enough pad. You'll find incontinence pads in your local drugstore. If you pass considerable amounts of uncontrolled urine, pick a weight that will hold about two hours' accumulation. Except for overnight use, it's better to keep to smaller pads and change often. This makes less visible bulging, protects your skin and other tissues from urine scald, and keeps you from getting stuck with a fortune's worth of pads when your situation improves. You can wear two pads on top of one another if you have no convenient way to carry spares. Only the outer pad need be attached to the retaining belt. Discard the inner pad when moist.

If you have mild incontinence, you'll find the "Maxi-" or "Minipads" sold for feminine hygiene much less expensive and more comfortable than pads made specifically for incontinence. You don't even need a belt or other device to support these; just stick them to the appropriate area of your underclothing.

STEP THREE: Powder moist areas when changing pads. Dusting powder helps keep skin and tissue that stays moist under the absorbent pad from becoming uncomfortable. Don't use heavily scented powders, since you can get a rash from the perfume they contain. You'll find all of the following, which are listed in order from most to least intensely drying, in the baby product section of your drugstore:

- Prickly heat powder
- Mexana®
- Diaprene® powder
- Talc (baby powder)

PRIME STRETCHER 3

*Relieve bladder infection or irritation with
fluids and diet.*

Burning pain on urination, need to void frequently, and cloudy,
smoky-looking urine generally come from bladder infection.
The bacteria that cause such infection can get into a man's
bladder only from his kidneys or bloodstream, so if you're a
man you should always see a doctor promptly about such
symptoms. Bacteria can get into a woman's bladder in two
other ways: through sexual activity, which can transport bacteria
up the urethra from the body surface into the bladder, and
from improper cleansing after a bowel movement.

STEP ONE: Prevent cystitis by choosing apt sex positions.
Would you believe that "honeymoon cystitis" strikes women
over forty as well as new brides? Looser tissues and
postmenopausal thinning of the vaginal wall let even moderate
sexual activity irritate the adjacent bladder. You can keep from
having this problem by avoiding sex positions that direct the
thrust of the penis forward, such as the woman's heels on the
man's shoulders. If you have had cystitis in the past, you might
go even farther and stick to such positions as the woman's
legs straight and the man straddling them, which direct thrust
toward the back of the vagina and away from the bladder.

STEP TWO: Cleanse aptly after bowel movements. The
easiest way to use toilet paper is to reach between your legs.
This approach unfortunately tends to drag soiled paper into
the vicinity of the urethral opening. You can avoid considerable
risk of cystitis by leaning forward, reaching around and wiping
one time only from front to rear with each piece of paper.

**STEP THREE: Drink extra fluid during periods of sexual
activity as a preventive measure, and as a first step in
treatment if urination starts to burn.** If you drink a lot of
fluid, you pass more urine. This washes bacteria out of your

bladder. Extra fluid intake during periods of sexual activity may prevent cystitis altogether by removing bacteria before they get a chance to invade your tissues. It also tips the balance toward self-cure if infection starts.

You'll find it easier to drink small quantities often—say a small juice glass every 15 minutes—than to choke down a full glass or more at once. Fruit juice, ginger ale, 7 Up®, and other no-caffeine, no-alcohol liquids seem most palatable.

STEP FOUR: Acidify your system by choice of foods and fluids. Most of the bacteria that cause cystitis make ammonia, which turns your urine alkaline (opposite of acid). Those bacteria then thrive in the alkaline environment.

If you eat and drink only materials that leave acid residue in your system, your urine will become more acidic and will neutralize the bacteria-produced alkali. This helps your body fight off the germs and heal itself. The foods and beverages

---

Foods That Acidify Your Urine

Meats, fish, and poultry. Shellfish. Eggs. Cheese. Peanuts and peanut butter.
Brazil nuts, filberts, walnuts, bacon.
Bread, especially whole wheat, cereal, crackers, pasta, rice.
Corn, lentils.
Plums, prunes, cranberries.
Cookies, uniced cake.

Foods to Avoid While Acidifying

Milk and dairy products (other than cheese).
Almonds, chestnuts, coconut.
All vegetables except corn and lentils.
Molasses.

---

listed in the box will acidify your system and help fight bladder infection.[1] Use it in conjunction with high fluid intake whenever burning on urination and frequency occur.

STEP FIVE: Decide when you need further help. Although mild cystitis usually yields to these measures promptly applied, symptoms sometimes persist. In that case, one of three things has usually happened:

1. You might have an underlying condition that caused the bladder infection in the first place. Kidney infection can cause no symptoms at its main site and still feed bacteria into the bladder. Bladder stones, ulcers, or tumors can make your bladder more prone to infection.

2. You might have encountered a particularly nasty kind of bacteria that you can't throw off without antibiotics.

3. You may have a condition that reduces your ability to fight infection, like diabetes.

Because all these conditions call for prompt medical treatment, you should see your doctor if

- Your urine looks pink or bloody.

- You get chills and fever or temperature over 100°F.

- You get pain or tenderness over the kidney area, which is located in the angle made by your lower ribs and spinal column.

- Symptoms persist over 48 hours.

---

[1] Some of the foods and fluids that you think of first when you want to build dietary acids actually leave alkaline rather than acid residues in your system. Citrus fruits and juices, for instance, are acid when you consume them, but the residues that appear in the urine are alkaline.

PRIME STRETCHER 4

Avoid cystocele and rectocele.

The walls between the bladder or rectum and the vagina can stretch and bulge. A cystocele or rectocele results—a bulging of the front or back wall of the vagina, which tends to become more prominent when straining at stool or with coughs and sneezes.

You can probably prevent cystocele and rectocele with these measures:

1. Heed any urge to urinate. An overfull bladder places strain on the tissues that keep the bladder wall from protruding into the vagina. Voiding promptly avoids this strain.
2. Vitamin C (ascorbic acid) strengthens the elastic and fibrous tissues of the bladder-vagina and rectum-vagina walls. If you note any tendency toward bulging when straining at stool, take 200 milligrams of ascorbic acid (obtainable without a prescription) daily.
3. Pelvic floor muscle exercises, discussed in Prime Stretcher 1, help strengthen the bladder-vagina wall.
4. Avoid constipation. See Chapter 6.
5. Lean forward and wrap your forearms in front of your knees during difficult bowel movements. This position directs bowel contents directly out of the rectum, while sitting upright directs thrust forward into the rectovaginal wall.

PRIME STRETCHER 5

Relieve prostate troubles with Sitz baths, ice packs, and pubic hair tugs.

If you're a man, your prostate gland can cause several kinds of trouble.

- Congestion from sexual deprival can cause low-back pain and sometimes difficulty starting the stream of urine.

- If the congestion comes from infection, you will usually have these symptoms plus burning discomfort toward the end of urination. You may also have poor quality erections or impotence. Some severe infections cause fever, muscular aching, and headache.

- Prostate enlargement can partially block passage of urine. You may have trouble starting the stream, dribbling at the end of urination, or need to void frequently (because you're not emptying your bladder when you urinate). With severe blockage, where you can't empty your bladder, it distends painfully.

- Prostate cancer can cause similar partial or total blockage.

STEP ONE: Fight congestion with sitz baths. Steady, dull pain in your low back unrelated to injury or strain quite often comes from prostate congestion. If so, you can usually get relief with sitz baths.

1. Run 4 inches of hot water into your tub. The temperature should be about 108°F if you have a candy or other accurate thermometer.

2. Sit in this pool with a towel wrapped around your shoulders. Sitting in hot water makes you perspire, and you'll need the towel to keep from getting chilled.

3. Occasionally replace some of the water with a freshly heated supply to maintain the temperature. Always check the temperature with your hand when adding hot water; immersed parts of your body become so used to the heat that you can burn yourself if you depend on their sensitivity. Keep the water level about the same—you're trying to spur extra circulation in the immersed parts, and the blood won't know where to go if most of your body is immersed.

4. Continue for about half an hour.

If your prostate has become infected, you need to see your doctor to get prescription-strength antibiotics. He will also draw pus out of the gland by massaging it (with one finger inside your rectum). Sitz baths will still be worthwhile, not only for relief of discomfort but also to increase flow of antibiotic-carrying blood through the gland.

STEP TWO: Ease urinary obstruction with ice or the pubic hair tug. You really should see a doctor whenever you can't pass your urine freely. Prompt care often gives lifelong cure if you have prostate or bladder cancer, so an immediate examination can be crucial to cure. Less serious causes are much more likely than cancer, though. Once you know that you don't have cancer, you'll probably put off surgery for a while.

When you have an enlarged prostate that you know isn't a cancer, you'll sometimes have a hard time starting the stream of urine. Three measures often help.

1. Turn on the water in the sink and let it flow. The sound of running water sometimes helps to relax the cut-off-the-stream muscle and makes it easier to void.

2. Apply cold applications to the crotch. Wrap crushed ice in a moist towel and hold against the crotch area for 5 minutes. This will often shrink the prostate enough that it ceases to block urine flow.

3. Pull out two or three pubic hairs. This rather extreme remedy causes reflex spasm of the arteries to the prostate, reducing its size temporarily. It may let you void when all other methods fail.

STEP THREE: Don't put off surgery too long. If your prostate blocks free passage of urine to the extent that your bladder doesn't empty fully, stagnant urine can readily become infected. And back pressure can do permanent damage to your kidneys.

If you have to get up at night more than twice to void, chances are that your bladder isn't emptying completely. At that point, you should consider having the obstructing gland pared back. Your urologist can do this through an instrument inserted through the penis, without a cutting operation. The procedure won't end your sex life: you'll ejaculate into your bladder instead of through the penis, but erection and sexual enjoyment will be unaffected.

CHAPTER 6

Free Yourself from Constipation, Hemorrhoids, and Hernias the Natural Way

You can make your bowel movements comfortable and regular through your choice of foods, by establishing a regular time for going to the bathroom and with other natural means. This stretches your prime in several crucial ways. It frees you of dependency on laxatives or cathartics and still keeps you clear of constipation, which (as the years go by) often cause more and more gas pains, bloating, and headache. It makes rectal miseries such as fissure and hemorrhoids much less likely. It even decreases your chances of having a hernia later.

Let's take a look at each of these effects, and how you can achieve them.

PRIME STRETCHER 1

Free yourself of dependency on laxatives.

If I could peek into your medicine chest, I could tell you almost instantly whether you have constipation. This is not because the remedies I see there show your need, but because many of the laxatives I might see actually cause that need to continue.

Irritant laxatives cause more constipation than any disease, disorder, stress, or bad habit. These laxatives work partly or wholly by irritating your bowel lining. A mildly irritated bowel weeps, moistening the stool, and making it easier to pass. Irritation also makes bowel muscles contract. A little extra muscle action moves material through your intestine more quickly, which gives prompt relief from constipation symptoms. But if the bowel muscle stays tight afterward, that holds back later passage. So any irritant laxative can cause (and frequently *does* cause) this vicious circle:

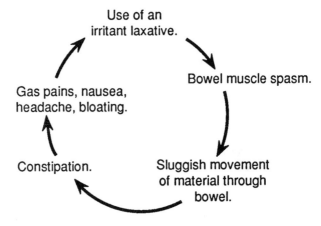

You can use the following method for establishing regular and natural elimination whether you've been taking laxatives or not. Past laxative use just makes it more important to take plenty of time going through the first four steps.

STEP ONE: Give up coffee, tea, cola, and other caffeine-containing drinks for life. These have no bulk, but they often increase bowel muscle spasm, increasing the harmful residual effect of irritant laxatives.

STEP TWO: Throw away all bowel function medicines except those listed in the box on the next page. Save the acceptable products for later use (in Step Five).

STEP THREE: Rest and soothe your bowel with a low-bulk diet. Picture your bowel constricted to half its normal size by irritation-induced spasm. The last thing it needs is extra bulk

---

Bowel Control Products for Occasional Use

Stool softeners
 Surfak®

Lubricants
 Petromul®
 Petrolagar®

Moist bulk producers
 Psillium seed
 Metamucil®
 Mucilose®

NOTE: Be sure these are "plain." Several are also marketed with added phenolpthalein or cascara, which makes them unsuitable.

---

inside its shrunken passageway! Yet that's what most natural food programs for constipation suggest: not just bulk but the dry, bowel-scraping bulk of bran! Those products have a place in constipation control, but not in the early stages. Until your bowel has been thoroughly soothed, you should avoid bran, whole wheat, and high-fiber cereals altogether.

When you stop taking laxatives, let your bowel rest and soothe away its spasm for the first two weeks. During this time, you can freely eat meat, dairy products, eggs and white or rye bread. Eat two normal servings of fruit or juice a day: one of lemon, orange, or grapefruit and one of bananas, pears, peaches, peeled apricots, baked apple, or strawberries. Also eat two servings of well-cooked peas, string beans, carrots, beets, spinach, tomato, or potato.

STEP FOUR: Use salt and soda or Fleet's® enemas if necessary for temporary relief during this stage. Whenever you have discomforts like headache, nausea and cramps, or whenever you go more than three days without a movement, use an enema for relief. A *salt and soda enema* (see description) works best.

As an alternate when you're away from home, a Fleet's Disposable Enema® (or one of its generic equivalents), available at your drugstore without prescription, generally gives prompt relief.

Salt and Soda Enema

Dissolve 1 teaspoonful of table salt and 2 teaspoonfuls of baking soda in 1 quart of lukewarm water. Place in an enema bag. Use the smallest enema tip. Lubricate well with petroleum jelly. Lie on your left side, and insert the tip just far enough that it stays. Gradually raise the enema bag until it is one to two feet above the level of the enema tip, and let the mixture flow in gently. If abdominal discomfort develops, lower the bag somewhat and gently knead the left lower portion of your abdomen with your free hand. When the enema has all run in, remove the tip and prepare for an evacuation. As soon as an urge develops, the enema is working fully: you need not try to hold back. (This is not true of the Fleet's® enema, which must be retained for several minutes to work effectively.)

You can make two adjustments in the enema routine.

- Change the volume to suit your own needs and comfort. If you feel that you need and could tolerate more volume, put a double amount in the enema bag and run in as much as you can comfortably absorb. If the 1-quart volume causes discomfort, use a Fleet's Disposable Enema® (or generic equivalent), which generally produces good evacuation with very little volume.

- If movements prove hard or massive, try *preliminary internal oiling.* Fleet's® makes an oil retention enema kit that is ideal for this purpose. As an alternative, you can put 2 ounces of warm olive oil in an infant or ear syringe, lubricate and insert the tip, then slowly squirt the oil into your rectum. After you concentrate on holding it for a few moments, the urge to defecate will pass. Retain the oil for half an hour; then use a salt and soda enema to produce evacuation.

STEP FIVE: Gradually increase moist bulk foods. After two weeks, all residual irritation from laxatives will be gone. You can start to work toward improved *fully natural* elimination by gradually building your consumption of *moist-bulk-producing* foods. At first, stick to the mild, never irritating fruits. Cautiously work in the more bowel-stimulating fruits like figs and dates after a week or two, going back to the milder ones if you get any bloating or discomfort.

Gentle Moist-bulk Producers

Stewed prunes	Currants
Cantaloupe	Applesauce
Honeydew melon	Plums
Persian melon	Cherries
Cranshaw melon	Berries
Raisins	

If movements remain difficult to pass, you can take one of the lubricating or softening medications mentioned. None of these speed the passage of material through your intestine, so each dose takes effect in about two days. Start with a tablespoonful twice a day of one of the liquids (or one pill or capsule twice a day). Adjust the dose up or down every three days until you find the minimum amount that leads to completely comfortable movements.

STEP SIX: Gradually add bran, oat bran, and fiber. After six weeks, you should have achieved comfortable elimination with the aid of only harmless lubricating or bulk-forming medicines. *Frequency of movements makes no difference at all!* Most people who go back to laxatives at this point have no gas pains, nausea, headache, hard-to-pass movements, or other true constipation symptoms. They just have smaller or less frequent stools than they think is right. *Stool bulk and frequency mean absolutely nothing!* The moist bulk you have eaten softens the stool, but doesn't provide much volume. As long as you have no digestive complaints and pass normal, sausage-shaped stools without discomfort, you're doing fine.

Now you can start adding dry-bulk foods. Try two slices of whole wheat or multigrain bread a day for three days. If this causes no gas, cramps, or stool hardness, increase to four slices (perhaps two as breakfast toast and two in a sandwich). If this causes no problems in three days, add breakfast cereal with bran or oat bran plus increased high-fiber vegetables like celery, carrots, turnips, and rutabagas.

You will find that eating these substances increases the bulk and frequency of your stools. Don't stop eating moist-bulk items, though; you still need them to keep stools soft. If you have no gas pains or cramps and can comfortably pass your stools without straining, cut back gradually on the *amount* of lubricating or stool-softening medication, but not on its *frequency.* Continue at least daily doses until you have cut to 1 teaspoonful or less daily.[1] Stay on this very small dose for a week before cutting it out altogether.

If you get cramps or hard-to-pass stools when you stop the medicine, go back on moderate amounts and increase your intake of moist-bulk-producing fruit. After a few weeks, try to taper off the medication again.

If you still don't achieve good natural elimination, start over with Steps One through Five, continue to omit bran and fiber, increase moist-bulk-producing fruits, and try reducing use of lubricating or stool-softening medications. You

---

[1] If you have been using a softener like Surfak® that comes in capsule form, you may need to switch to a liquid lubricant like Petromul® during the tapering-off phase. You can't cut the capsules, so you can't take decreasing doses.

may be one of the none-too-rare people who just don't tolerate dry bulk.

STEP SEVEN: Develop a habit time and routine. Like other digestive functions, bowel function readily becomes linked with certain circumstances. Just as your mouth waters when you smell turkey, your bowel associates its function with other stimuli or events. If you pick a convenient time (preferably after a meal, when body rhythms already lean toward a movement) and spend 10 minutes or so on the toilet every day, you will soon find your body cooperating. Adding other routine and relaxing activities, such as reading the funny papers or doing the crossword puzzle, reinforces the process.

If you establish a habit time by following it rigidly for two or three weeks, you will find that it not only helps you to plan your day but also helps you to maintain natural elimination.

PRIME STRETCHER 2

Ease rectal itching.

You need more rest as the years go by. That means more sitting, which often also means trapped moisture in the rectal area. Ordinary methods of cleansing after a bowel movement leave behind irritants and bacteria (especially if bulging hemorrhoids make thorough cleansing more difficult), which can invade moisture-softened skin. Rectal itching, with or without visible skin changes, often follows.

If the area isn't visibly inflamed or sensitive, changed cleansing methods often control the problem.

STEP ONE: Replace toilet paper friction with gentler, more effective cleansing methods. My Johns Hopkins bacteriology professor used to say that if feces were red we would live in a crimson world. He used this rather repellent statement to point up the fact that moist paper presents no barrier whatever to bacteria. He might also have explained that paper removes very few irritants or germs, and that even the softest varieties scratch and scrape irritated skin.

Ordinarily, the harm done by inadequate cleansing doesn't justify getting out of step with the rest of American society and using a different approach. Just use the paper and wash your hands thoroughly afterward. But when itching shows that bacteria and irritants have invaded your tissues, use a different cleansing technique.

- Keep a liquid soap dispenser, a bottle of rubbing alcohol, some talc or cornstarch, and some cotton balls handy in the bathroom. Fill the washbasin partly with warm water before you sit down to have a bowel movement. When you have finished, dip a cotton ball in the warm water, squirt a drop of liquid soap on it, and use it to cleanse the rectal area. Repeat two or three times, until the ball remains reasonably clean.

- Use two or three sopping-wet cotton balls to rinse away any soap remnant.

STEP TWO: Use a wick, alcohol, and talc to control itch-causing seepage. Small amounts of rectal moisture normally tend to seep out through the anal opening. This bacteria- and irritant-laden material is a major cause of rectal itching.

One of the best ways to control this seepage is by inserting a wisp of cotton into the canal. Pull a cotton ball apart into two roughly equal halves. Stretch one half until it is about 2 inches long. Smooth it over the tip of your index finger and insert it into the rectal opening just far enough that it will stay in place. This works in two ways: by causing reflex contraction of the muscle, which seals off the opening, and by acting as a wick. (If you have large hemorrhoids, you may need to use the whole cotton ball and insert it a bit farther into the rectum to keep it in place.)

Unless open scratch marks make alcohol sting, it also helps to sponge the area with rubbing alcohol on one cotton ball. Dry with more cotton balls; then dust the area with talc or cornstarch.

If scratch marks or raw tissue make alcohol sting, you need further soothing treatment. Get Cortaid® cream (or its generic equivalent) at your drugstore and apply a thin coat three times a day.

STEP THREE: Try malt soup extract. If itching persists after giving this technique a ten-day trial, you can change the bacterial content of your stools by taking malt soup extract. You'll find this in the infant care section of your drugstore, since it is usually used to modify baby formula to get rid of diaper rash. Take 1 tablespoonful either mixed with cereal or stirred in water with each of your three meals. Since malt soup extract needs several days to work, you should try it for at least a week before deciding whether it will help you.

PRIME STRETCHER 3

Cure rectal splits and fissures by prompt action.

Passage of a hard stool will often split the skin at the rectal opening. You will then feel pain immediately after each movement, when your control muscle closes off the opening and presses on the sore spot.

Unless you take prompt steps to heal this split, hard scar tissue will form at its base. This inelastic tissue will hold the edges of the split apart and keep it from healing. A split that can't heal itself is called a "fissure in ano" and requires surgery.

Prompt apt home care can prevent all that. As soon as you realize that a split has occurred, take these steps:

STEP ONE: Take medication and introduce oil to keep stools soft and easily passed while the split heals. Take a tablespoonful of Metamucil® twice a day. Mix this with a full glass of water, and drink another glass of water immediately after each dose. (Metamucil® works by soaking up a lot of moisture within your intestine, so you need to provide a lot of extra liquid to make it work well.)

Get a 2-ounce all-rubber ear syringe from your drugstore. At bedtime, fill it with olive or mineral oil. Lubricate and insert the soft rubber tip into your rectum, being careful to avoid pressure on the sore split spot. Slowly squeeze the oil into your bowel cavity. Pull out the syringe, retaining the oil. Sleep in panties or underpants with a feminine hygiene pad stuck inside in case any oil seeps out. If you go two days without a movement, replace this 2-ounce oil application with a Fleet's Oil Retention Enema® at bedtime. Unless a movement has occurred by 10 A.M. the following day, take a salt and soda enema with one possible modification in technique:

If you find that the usual enema tip causes discomfort pressing against the split, get a small, soft rubber catheter. Insert the hard enema tip into the open end of the catheter, lubricate the other end (the blunt one with one or more holes at its side), and insert it 2 or 3 inches into your lower bowel.

STEP TWO: Use ointment to soothe the split. Put a glob of zinc oxide ointment on the tip of your ear syringe when you take your nightly oil application treatment. Apply the ointment in the same way (without the oil) twice during the day.

If you get persistent pain after movements, use Surfacaine Ointment® or Nupercainal® every eight hours for relief. (You can get either with a rectal applicator.)

STEP THREE: Relieve spasm of the bowel control muscle with heat or suppositories. At first, you may need to apply hot wet towels to the area, changing them to keep them hot for 10 minutes, after each bowel movement. Alternately, you can take hot sitz baths.

When the pain becomes mild, suppositories may give more convenient relief. If you have hemorrhoids along with the split, insert an Anusol® suppository every 12 hours. Always unwrap and insert suppositories blunt end first. Anusol® will help shrink swollen tissues. If you have no noticeable hemorrhoid bulges in the area, Wyanoid® suppositories will work better. You can buy either type at your drugstore without a prescription.

If the split hasn't healed after four weeks, you should see your doctor. A scar tissue base will almost always have formed by this time, making an operation necessary. With today's measures for pain relief, such surgery won't cause the pain you might expect.

PRIME STRETCHER 4

Prevent hemorrhoids or soothe them with sitz baths, ointments or suppositories.

Suspect hemorrhoids if

- You feel a soft protrusion near the anal opening when cleansing after a movement.
- You get itching or discomfort or one of the protrusions becomes swollen and sore.
- You notice blood on the toilet paper or on the surface of the stool. Hemorrhoids often lie within rather than outside the anal opening. In this case, you will not feel any bulge, and bleeding will often be the only symptom. *Any kind of rectal bleeding deserves a doctor's attention since it could come from a tumor that will become life-threatening if not promptly treated.* Don't be too alarmed, though: the less serious conditions outnumber the serious ones better than 10 to 1.

STEP ONE: Slow the growth of early hemorrhoids (and often let them heal themselves) by avoiding actions that build abdominal pressure like straining at stool, improper lifting, or uncontrolled cough. Hemorrhoids form when a vein in the anal area becomes engorged. The veins in this area connect to two different parts of your circulation: the main channel by which blood returns to your heart and the system of veins within your abdomen that ends in your liver. If the pressure in one system becomes higher than that in the other, blood detours through the hemorrhoidal veins and they enlarge to handle the extra flow.

What increases the pressure in the inside-the-abdomen system of veins?

- A pregnancy, in which the growing baby takes up part of the limited space within the abdomen, increasing the pressure on all the contents of that enclosed space
- Improper lifting, when you stop breathing and grunt
- Straining at stool
- Coughing
- Liver disorders, which block the flow of blood out of the other end of this vein system

You can take effective action against all but the first and last of these.

1. Keep breathing in and out instead of holding your breath and grunting when you lift. Watch the Olympic weight lifters and you'll see that they keep breathing evenly throughout the action. That lets pressure dissipate through the diaphragm. They do this mainly to prevent hernia (which we'll discuss shortly), but the same technique will help you heal small hemorrhoids or keep them from happening in the first place.

2. Avoid straining at stool by developing healthy elimination with this section's Prime Stretcher 1.

3. Keep effective cough medicines in your medicine cabinet and use them whenever you're coughing hard. Cough control can save you from a lot of later trouble with hemorrhoids and hernia. (In the days when we couldn't cure tuberculosis, it often made victims cough for months or years. Those patients got more hernias and hemorrhoids than any manual laborer, including ditch diggers and warehousemen.)

STEP TWO: Control mild discomfort with ointments or suppositories. Mild hemorrhoidal discomfort comes mainly from surfaces rubbing together and becoming irritated. Use zinc oxide ointment (obtainable at your drugstore without a prescription) twice a day to soothe those areas. Put a dab on the nearby skin and let it warm to body temperature for a minute or so. Then you can spread it more easily. Cotton underclothing will absorb any excess, which will wash out readily.

Anusol® or Wyanoid® suppositories (also nonprescription) may give further relief. Unwrap and insert a suppository blunt end first after or between bowel movements, not more often than every twelve hours.

STEP THREE: Soothe clotted hemorrhoids with ointments and hot towels or sitz baths. When a hemorrhoid swells and becomes very tender, the swollen vein at its core has stopped up with a clot. Heat helps your body to carry that clot away. Hot towels or a sitz bath give temporary relief and actually speed healing.

Apply a thin coat of Nupercainal® or Surfacaine® ointment after the heat treatment for further relief.

If the hemorrhoid becomes larger than the tip of your thumb, you will probably want more rapid relief than home measures can give. Your doctor can make a tiny cut into the hemorrhoid and pop the clot out, which makes it feel better immediately and speeds the healing process.

PRIME STRETCHER 5

Prevent or deal with hernia.

Your abdominal wall has a thin elastic lining layer inside its firm layers of muscle and connective tissue. The firm layers have some gaps, where certain structures penetrate. Weak spots include

- A man's groin, where tubes carrying sperm from the testes penetrate

- The belly button where crucial blood vessels connected your circulation with your mother's before birth

- Any surgical incisions

- The portion of your diaphragm through which your esophagus passes en route from the chest to the abdomen

STEP ONE: Help diaphragmatic hernia by raising the head of your bed. Dealing with the last variety first, suspect a diaphragmatic hernia if you get heartburn in the middle of the night, especially if you are a bit heavy for your height. You may also note black, tarry stools (from fully digested blood: if your stomach wall pushes up into your chest cavity, the constricting band where it penetrates your diaphragm occasionally causes internal bleeding).

You will need X rays to be sure what has gone wrong, so you will probably get some medications from your physician. In addition to any medicines he gives you, I strongly recommend two measures:

- Lose weight. A certain proportion of excess fat in your body lies in the omentum, a flap of tissue within your abdomen. Shedding even a few pounds makes this organ shrink and makes more room inside your abdominal cavity. This often reduces the upward pressure against your diaphragm and may keep a diaphragmatic hernia from giving much trouble.

- Raise the head of your bed. Buy two 4-inch by 4-inch blocks 6 inches or 8 inches in length. Nail a curtain rod ring to the tops so that your bed coaster won't roll off the edges. Perch the head of your bedstead on the blocks. If you want to raise only one side of the bed, you can buy a large triangular pad that extends from the top of the bed to waist level (available at Penney's and other stores).

STEP TWO: Avoid emergency surgery with other hernias by using ice and home means of dealing with strangulation. If a gap in the supporting muscle tissue develops at any of the other points mentioned, the elastic lining layer bulges into the gap. Any increased pressure inside the abdomen then expands this bulge, like the bubble one can blow in well-chewed bubble gum. Some organs within the abdomen, such as intestine, hang free enough to work their way into any such hollow bulge. When any organ that belongs in your abdomen protrudes through its muscular wall, you have a hernia, also called a rupture.

The measures advised in Prime Stretcher 4's Step One to avoid hemorrhoids also help to ward off hernia. Breathing constantly while lifting, developing proper elimination, and controlling coughing will usually keep you clear of this condition.

If you get a hernia as large as a baseball, it almost certainly will contain a loop of intestine. This will work its way down through the narrow gap in your abdomen's muscular wall into the larger hollow space within the hernia's bulge. Then the narrow gap can act like a string around your intestine, cutting off flow of material in it. The trapped tissue then will swell, cutting off its own circulation.

That is how a hernia "strangulates." Once it gets to this stage, emergency surgery is the only answer, and the need to repair or remove the damaged segment of intestine makes the operation dangerous. The risk and discomfort of repairing the hernia before it strangulates are much less than such an emergency operation involves.

I never advise patients with a hernia to hold it in place with a truss. Such devices make you more comfortable, but actually increase the risk: if any intestine works its way under the truss, pressure from the device itself kicks off the process of strangulation.

If you get a hernia, strangulation may occur before you realize that your condition needs repair. If so, you may get cramps in your abdomen from intestinal obstruction without much tenderness in the hernia area itself. If you can get the trapped intestine back out of the hernia into the abdominal cavity *promptly* you may avoid the need for emergency surgery. First try to work the hernia's contents back into their proper place with gentle pressure. If you can't do that, fill a plastic bag with chipped ice, wrap it in a wet towel, and apply to the area where the hernia originates for 5 minutes, then try again. If you still can't empty the hernia sac (and it is in your groin), chill it again and get a helper to use this maneuver:

Take off your shoes. Stand on the bed near its foot. Have the hernia victim lie on his back and stretch his legs straight up, supporting his hips with his hands, with his elbows pressed against the bed. Now hold his legs against your chest with both your arms, and jump up and down on the bed as if you were on a trampoline.

This procedure will often work the hernia's contents back into their proper place. *If these measures don't completely empty the hernia, go to a doctor or emergency room right away.* Organs trapped within a hernia lose their circulation and need to be removed within a few hours, making the necessary operation more and more extensive and dangerous. *You should not stick with home measures for more than an hour or two at most.*

CHAPTER 7

Save Those Teeth, Spare Those Gums!

Sound teeth help you to stretch your prime in several ways.

- Your teeth help to keep you from looking old. Not only your grin but your facial contours depend on sound teeth, without which you develop sunken cheeks and an altered jaw line.

- If you become self-conscious about these appearance changes, poor or missing teeth can impair crucial parts of your interplay with people.

- Good teeth make a huge difference to your digestion. Chewing breaks up chunks of food so that digestive juices can get at every particle. It also mixes saliva, which contains an enzyme crucial to digestion of starch, through each bite. If you can't chew well, you usually get gas cramps and often nausea or heartburn from a great many foods.

You can take several steps in your own home to make tooth loss less likely.

PRIME STRETCHER 1

*Fight periodontitis by removing irritants
from tooth-gum slots.*

When you first learned to brush your teeth, *preventing cavities* was your main purpose. By age forty, you need to change the emphasis. *Periodontitis* causes much more tooth loss than cavities in fully mature adults.

This disorder starts with inflammation of the gums adjacent to the teeth. Pus pockets burrow down into the gums beside the emerging tooth roots. Infection then extends into the bony tissue adjacent to the roots, making teeth loose. A loose tooth damages its roots further, and the tooth ultimately is lost.

This whole process starts when food particles get into the space between the gum margin and the tooth. If irritating or bacteria-feeding food fragments stay long enough to cause tissue to swell, they get caught between the swollen gum tissue and the tooth. Irritation goes on and on, making the gums tender and easily injured. The first noticeable sign of this disorder is usually "pink toothbrush"—bleeding caused by brushing or other contact your tissues should readily withstand.

STEP ONE: Brush differently after age forty to prevent periodontitis. To clean irritants out of the gum-tooth crease, you should brush after each meal, using a special technique.

1. Get a toothbrush with very fine, soft bristles. Stiff bristles cause discomfort when applied to tender gum tissue and will not flex sufficiently to work into the gum-tooth crease (see the next steps). Also obtain antiplaque toothpaste if you aren't already using it.

2. Draw your lips back so that you can see the surfaces of your front teeth. Hold your toothbrush so that the bristles are perpendicular to the middle of your front teeth. Press back against the tooth and note how the bristles flare out so that those at the margin lie almost parallel with the tooth surface.

3. Maintaining enough pressure to keep the bristles flared, move the brush slowly toward the gum line. Note how the flared bristle tips slide along the tooth surface and disappear under the gum edge. *This is the action you need to clean out the gum-tooth creases.*

4. Using antiplaque toothpaste, brush the outside and inside surfaces of each tooth by pressing the bristles into its center and using circular movement to both polish the tooth and work the flared bristle tips into the gum-tooth creases. Always keep the head of the brush parallel with the tooth surfaces, getting the bristles into the gum-tooth crease by pressing harder to make more flare instead of by angling the brush. Be especially thorough in brushing the outer surfaces of your lower molars. (Possibly because your main salivary glands empty into your mouth at this point, keeping the gum tissues constantly overmoist, this area is the usual starting point of periodontitis.)

5. After your main meal, floss to remove food particles from between your teeth.

STEP TWO: Use your fingertip instead of your toothbrush for gum massage. When you were younger, you were probably taught to start each brush stroke on your gums over the roots of your teeth. This technique doesn't get the bristles down into the gum line pouches, so you should replace it with the method described in Step One. But that doesn't mean that you should abandon gum massage altogether. Once a day you should follow tooth brushing with fingertip gum massage. Press the tip of your right index finger firmly into the gum tissue high above the outer surface of your left upper molars. Maintaining pressure, slide your finger down onto the teeth. Move your finger forward a bit and repeat. Continue until you have massaged down over the outer gum-tooth margin on all upper teeth. Being careful not to start far enough back to cause a gag reflex, follow a similar technique on the inside surfaces, then on the lower teeth.

Other Causes of Bleeding Gums

Medications
    Anticoagulants, including Aspirin, Persantine®, Coumarin®,
       and Dicumerol®
    Dilantin®
    Tumor fighters
Vitamin C deficiency
Rare diseases
    Aplastic anemia
    Purpura
    Leukemia

Massage helps in two ways. It stimulates circulation and also helps you to detect early irritation. Tenderness or traces of blood on your fingertip usually show early periodontitis. The accompanying box indicates some other causes of bleeding gums that might confuse the picture.

PRIME STRETCHER 2

*Treat early gum inflammation with
mouthwash, massage, and special flossing.*

As soon as you note gum tenderness or traces of blood on either your toothbrush or your massaging fingertip, step up your irritant removal program.

STEP ONE: Use saltwater mouthwash to remove bacteria. After each meal and before brushing your teeth, dissolve half a teaspoonful of table salt in a glass of warm water. Take a mouthful and swish it around between your teeth. Spit it out and take another mouthful. Continue until you have used up all the salt solution. *This removes bacteria just as thoroughly as any antiseptic.*

STEP TWO: Massage more often. Massage your gums using the foregoing technique *three times* daily instead of once. This increases blood supply and helps to fight infection.

STEP THREE: Use a special flossing technique to remove irritants. Take a long piece of dental floss. Wrap its end around your right index finger. Leave about a 2-inch gap, then wrap it around your left index finger. Press the segment between your two index fingers down between your two rearmost left lower molars. Push both your fingers toward the back of your head so that the floss wraps halfway around the back tooth. Work it up and down two or three times. Pull your fingers toward the front of your head so that the floss wraps halfway around the second tooth. Work it up and down. Use the same technique with the floss between the second and third lower molars, then with it between each other pair of teeth in your mouth. (You can't really work the floss into the gum-tooth crease, but food fragments trapped there often extend above the margin enough to be displaced with this technique.)

If gums remain tender or bleed easily after following these three steps for a week, see your dentist or periodontist (a dentist specializing in care of this particular disorder).

PRIME STRETCHER 3

Consider implants.

If you lose (or have lost) the teeth necessary to make fixed bridges work, you need to choose between full or partial dentures and implants. Implants have great advantages.

- They usually last for life.

- By letting you chew anything and everything more thoroughly, they help keep you clear of digestive miseries.

- You avoid "denture breath" and annoying cleansing and inserting routines.

You do not need an implant to replace every single lost tooth. A dentist can anchor a fixed bridge between two implants or from a sound tooth to an implant.

Since the tissue into which the implant fits has less nerve supply than a tooth root, you'll have less discomfort than you might expect if you have an implant. Under some circumstances, Medicare and ordinary (not specifically dental) insurance covers all or part of the expense.

PRIME STRETCHER 4

Minimize the effect of lost teeth with gum care, food preparation, and starch digestants.

When I was first in practice, I had patients who had full dentures while still in their twenties.

"Why get them fixed over and over, *then* get them pulled?" one patient asked.

After treating both that patient and dozens of other denture wearers for digestive miseries, I can easily answer that question. Elephants die when they lose their teeth. People just suffer gas pains, heartburn, nausea, and constipation. Dentures may be better than nothing, but they're not nearly as effective as your original teeth.

Don't get into this situation if you can avoid it. But if you do, you can minimize the harmful effects on your gums and your digestive system with the following methods.

STEP ONE: Keep gums healthy with massage, and prompt care for sores. Dentures put your gums in a cast. Just as your arm or leg withers when kept motionless and inactive, gums shrink. Then dentures fit poorly and need to be relined.

You can keep this change to a minimum. Buy a teething ring in the infant department of your drugstore. After removing your dentures at night, chomp hard on the ring, moving it between each bite until your entire gum surface has been stimulated.

If this process reveals any tender area, look at it carefully. You will usually find a shiny, wet whitish patch. This indicates pus lying in a gap in the surface layer of the gum or palate, usually from erosion by viral or bacterial infection. This will heal more quickly if you apply *10 percent silver nitrate solution.* You can obtain this from your drugstore without a prescription. Use a cotton-tipped applicator, moistening only the very tip with the solution. Touch only the affected area, since the silver nitrate will harm normal tissue. Apply this only once, and only when the sore has developed within 24 hours. *Keep silver nitrate in a safe place and away from the medicine chest, since it is very poisonous.*

Prompt silver nitrate application usually helps sores to heal within two or three days. In the meanwhile (or if you missed the boat by not applying the silver nitrate within the first 24 hours) apply Gly-oxide®, a solution of dehydrated glycerine that you can obtain at your drugstore without a prescription. Use the applicator tip of the container or apply with the handle end of your toothbrush.

Never apply silver nitrate to an area more than once. If the sore fails to heal promptly or recurs, see your dentist right away. Also, don't apply silver nitrate to leathery-looking or long-lasting white patches. These need prompt professional care.

STEP TWO: Cook vegetables until soft, meat until tender, but don't overdo the chopping and grinding. You can overdo the business of substituting a grinder, food processor, or overused knife and fork for thorough chewing. The chewing process not only chops up food, but also mixes starch-digesting saliva through it. If you reduce food to mush, you tend to swallow it directly. That leaves the starches totally undigested, and leads to gas cramps and bloating.

If your dentures don't allow thorough mastication of firm foods, chew each bite ten times (even if it's soft or you've already chopped it up) until you break the food-bolting habit. You will usually find that this improves your digestion considerably.

STEP THREE: Take starch digestants if necessary. Tooth troubles accumulate so gradually that you don't always know what they are doing to your digestion and your freedom to eat various foods. If you wear dentures and find yourself limiting your food choice to avoid indigestion, or if your dentures just don't let you comfortably chomp away until you've mixed saliva through every bite, try starch digestants. You'll need a prescription for these, and your doctor will probably want you to take stomach X rays first (to make sure you don't have a more serious cause for your indigestion than inadequate chewing). They do work reasonably well and keep you from having to restrict your food choices. (It's almost impossible to avoid starches in anything approaching a normal diet.)

Sarah K. had dropped out of almost all her social activities because she felt embarrassed. She had gotten where she passed gas and belched almost continually and just couldn't control it. She didn't really suffer much pain—just an occasional mild cramp—but the constant bloating and gas passage was ruining her life.

Sarah had lost all her teeth and wore full upper and lower dentures. The upper had become quite loose, making it difficult for her to chew. As a temporary measure, I prescribed starch digestants for her, explaining that if they worked it would almost prove that poor chewing had caused her problem. The gas improved considerably, although it didn't disappear completely. Sarah had her dentist reline her plates, chewed every bite ten times, and continued the starch digestants. The gas disappeared entirely. She gradually decreased the medication over a period of three weeks and found that she could keep the problem under control with thorough chewing alone.

CHAPTER
8

How to Keep Your Vision Sharp

Getting older causes some perfectly normal but aggravating changes in your vision. Let's review them.

PRIME STRETCHER 1

Compensate for aging eyes with reading glasses, large-print books, Polaroid® glasses, and special lighting.

As the years go by, the crystalline lens inside your eye loses its elasticity. By your mid-forties, you can no longer focus on near objects by changing the shape of your eye's lens. At this point, you need reading glasses or bifocals.

STEP ONE: Buy reading glasses in your local drugstore, if you can in your state. Although some states outlaw drugstore reading glasses, no one claims that they hurt your eyes. (The argument against them is that you should see a doctor whenever your vision changes.) Reading glasses come in various strengths from 1.0 to 4.0 or more diopters, and with various-length temples (the things that fit over your ears) from 32 to 40 millimeters (mm.). You can try various sizes and strengths to find those that let you read fine print at a comfortable and convenient distance (usually 12 to 15 inches).

These glasses have a big cost advantage over prescription lenses. The ones I own have exactly the right correction, but cost less than one-fourth what an optician wanted for made-to-order ones. But ready-made glasses also have several disadvantages, which may or may not apply to *you* (and may or may not be easily overcome).

- Drugstore reading glasses correct only for focusing. If you need any other kind of correction (e.g., for astigmatism), they won't help.

- Both the right and left lenses match, but your eyes may differ. (You may be able to find "Granny glasses" that are rimless at the top. If one pair corrects one eye and a different pair corrects the other eye, you can usually dissolve the glue from the right lens of each pair with nail polish remover, trade lenses, and use craft cement to glue the replacement into the frame with the correct left lens.)

- You may need to bend the temples to make them fit better. Pick glasses with metal temples to make this easier. If they have plastic pads in areas that you need to bend, immerse those portions in hot water (about 140°F) for 5 minutes before bending them to keep from cracking the plastic.

If your vision has been good without glasses, you will probably find that you need about 1.5 diopter readers at about age forty-five. You will need slightly stronger ones in your fifties, perhaps 2.5 diopters. As you get older, you may get "second sight"; aging changes your eyeball, and may alter the focus of your eye's lens system so that you can read with weaker and weaker glasses.

You'll probably find that the weakest lenses that give clear vision prove to be most convenient. You can still see well up close with somewhat stronger lenses, but *only* up close: they make objects a bit farther out much more blurred.

If you have previously been nearsighted or farsighted, you may need considerably different strength lenses—perhaps a maximum of 1.0 diopter if you've been nearsighted and as much as 4.0 diopters if you've been farsighted. If you have astigmatism or if one of your eyes differs considerably from the other, you will need to get prescription bifocals or trifocals.

STEP TWO: Shift home and office lighting as you age. The crystalline lens inside each of your eyes ultimately fogs slightly from age alone. This makes it hard for you to see clearly in dim light. At the same time, the center of those lenses may become opaque, so that your vision becomes poorer when your pupils contract in very bright light, making all the light that enters your eye travel through the center of each lens.

Fortunately, you can compensate for these changes with a different lighting arrangement. While your eyes do better when you're young if everything in your field of vision has about the same level of illumination, aging eyes have different requirements. A dim background helps keep your pupils open so that light can detour around the central opacity, while bright light on the small area where you are reading or working helps you overcome fogging.

You can get self-contained reflectorized spotlight bulbs at any hardware store. Try reading in an otherwise dimly lit room with a spotlight shining directly on your book. If the lens changes of age alone have cut your vision, you'll probably find that this arrangement lets you read much more easily.

Incidentally, your library probably has a section of large-type books. Many of my older patients find these much more relaxing to read. Why not give them a try?

STEP THREE: Fight glare with light-colored Polaroid® glasses. The same fogging of your eyes' crystalline lenses that makes you need brighter light on your work also diffuses glare as it enters your eyes and makes it much more annoying. That's why driving at night often becomes such a trial as the years go by.

Light that bounces off a level surface, such as a highway, has different qualities from light that comes directly from an ordinary source. All the light waves in bouncing light tend to be parallel with the surface from which they have bounced, which makes glare "polarized light." A film of Polaroid® has a very fine grid that does not let horizontal polarized light waves penetrate. While most Polaroid® sunglasses also have dark tinting, the dark tint isn't necessary for glare exclusion. If you can find a very light pair of Polaroid® glasses (or shields which attach to your regular glasses), you may find they make night driving much more safe and comfortable.

STEP FOUR: Don't let floaters, black specks, and scintillating streaks bother you. Three somewhat worrisome conditions frequently affect your eyes after age forty. These cause temporary and variable changes only and generally cause no permanent visual impairment.

Floaters make you see moving black dots, generally out of the corner of your eye. If your house didn't have screens, you probably wouldn't even notice these: you would just think a fly was buzzing around.

Most floaters come from dense clumps of cells in the clear globe of gel that fills your eyeball. These change position with eye movement (which is why they're called "floaters"). If one happens to work its way into the center of your visual field so that it distracts you when you are reading, you can usually get it out of the way by looking rapidly up, then down, then up.

The first time you notice a floater, use this technique to see if it moves. If it remains stationary after repeated rapid eye movements, it isn't a floater. Consider it a "stationary black spot."

Stationary black spots have a different cause. These come from age-related shrinkage of the clear globe of gel inside your eyeball. If this pulls away from the retina, its inner surface bounces light away before you perceive it and you seem to see a black speck. This speck will always be in the same place, although it gets lost in the background most of the time so that you only become conscious of it when you look at a blank page, plain white-painted wall or the like.

You don't need to worry about these specks as long as only one or two appear at a time and they don't increase in size. That's what usually happens. Very rarely a number of specks will appear in the same area within a short time, sometimes accompanied by a sensation of flashing light. These signs sometimes mean that the shrinking globe of clear gel has torn the retina or pulled it loose from its backing. If the retina drops away farther from its moorings, you might see a veil fall over a portion of your visual field in one eye.

You should get prompt attention from an eye doctor if any of these signs make you suspect retinal separation. The doctor can use a laser to tack the retina painlessly back in place and preserve vision.

Scintillating streaks appear simultaneously in both eyes. You see a pattern that looks like a flowing river of tiny black dots seen from an airplane. Sometimes this pattern will start near the center of your visual field and gradually move outward until it disappears. This process might last as much as 20 minutes if you take no countermeasures, but always disappears with no residual visual damage.

This is known as "ophthalmic migraine," which is a bad and frightening name for a condition that never becomes more than a slight nuisance. It is due to a brief spasm of a blood vessel in the part of your brain that receives vision signals.

A simple home remedy greatly shortens the duration of these attacks. Just hold every other breath as long as you can. This allows carbon dioxide, which you normally clear out of your system in expired air, to accumulate in your bloodstream. Carbon dioxide fights blood vessel spasm, so breath-holding usually will shorten ophthalmic migraine attacks to 5 minutes or less.

PRIME STRETCHER 2

Recognize and deal with impaired vision due to changed water balance in your system.

The first patient who made me aware of the effect of the body's water balance on vision had severe premenstrual edema. Thelma P. would suddenly gain seven or eight pounds of water weight every month a few days before her menstruation, then get back to her previous size a few days later. Along with two complete wardrobes, she had two pairs of glasses, because her vision also changed with the cycle. When Thelma was treated to keep from accumulating extra water in her system, she also found that the weaker glasses corrected her vision all the time.

I've seen this same effect in other patients who either had disorders or took medications that affected their water balance. Along with premenstrual edema, the most common disorders causing this visual variation are diabetes and nephritis. Some of the medications commonly used for high blood pressure, heart disease, and kidney disorders also have this effect.

Sometimes the underlying condition can be cured or a different medication used to control it. Otherwise, most patients breathe a sigh of relief when they learn that they don't have a serious eye disorder and they can buy pairs of stronger and weaker glasses.

PRIME STRETCHER 3

*Keep wind, wind-blown particles and
dryness from damaging your eyes.*

You can almost tell which of your friends has spent a lot of time in the outdoors by looking for yellowish triangular bumps just beside the inner edges of their corneas (the clear windows at the front of the eyes). Wind or windborne particles can cause these so-called phlectenules. Sometimes they will extend partway across the cornea, interfering with vision unless surgically removed.

You can almost always prevent this unsightly condition with two simple measures.

STEP ONE: Avoid or shelter your eyes from rapidly moving air. Remember the goggles airmen used to wear when flying in an open cockpit? No pilot would have flown without them, because wind and dust would not only make his eyes water and impair vision but also ultimately damage his eyes.

An automobile, snowmobile, or speedboat travels a lot faster than those early planes, but many riders just let the wind buffet them. Most people just don't seem to think of *air* through which they are moving as identical with *wind*. But when the air blasts your eyeballs, there's just no difference.

Usually you will be able to keep out of heavy airstreams just by using windshields or closing windows. But if you can't, either skier's goggles or wrap-around sunglasses will keep down wind damage.

STEP TWO: Get grit or cinders out of your eyes promptly. When anything irritating flies into your eye, take these steps immediately:

1. *Don't rub!* Pressure through your eyelid mashes any dust or cinders between your eyeball and your eyelid. Whichever the particles dig into, they're harder to dislodge and more irritating mashed into tissue than they would be loose.

2. Close your eye gently and place the tip of your index finger over your eyelashes, catching them against the top of your cheekbone.

3. Slide your finger, with the trapped lashes and underlying skin, down along your cheekbone. This pulls your eyelid away from your eyeball and makes a pocket in which tears can accumulate.

4. Let the tears accumulate inside your pulled-down eyelid for a few seconds.

5. Snap your eye open without moving your fingertip. This will usually leave the particles loose in the pool of tears inside your pulled-down lower lid.

6. Release the lower lid. The particle will usually float out with the accumulated teardrops.

If you still feel something in your eye after this maneuver, you probably have a particle imbedded in your tissues. A helper can usually get this out for you with this technique:

1. Assemble a small, long blunt object such as a lead pencil or a small key and a soft, absorbent object such as the corner of a handkerchief. A cotton-tipped applicator (Q-tip®) will fulfill both roles.

2. First, get your helper to search for the cinder under your lower lid. If it is there, touching it with the handkerchief tip or cotton-tipped applicator will usually remove it.

3. Next, get your helper to look carefully in good light for a black speck on the cornea. Any particle that has imbedded itself in the cornea needs prompt removal by a doctor (not necessarily a specialist—most general practitioners and emergency room physicians can remove such objects).

4. If the particle isn't in either of these places, it is almost certainly caught in the lining of your upper eyelid. Look down without closing your eye. Have your helper grasp your upper lid's lashes between his or her thumb and forefinger. He or she should then press the side of the tip of the blunt object against your eyelid about an eighth of an inch from the lid margin. By pulling the lashes forward while pressing back in this way, he or she can flip the soft half-inch pad of gristle that stiffens the margin of the lid down across the pupil. By stretching the skin of the lid slightly from the sides, your helper can keep the gristle from flipping back while finding the particle and dabbing at it with the corner of the handkerchief or cotton-tipped applicator. Once the particle is gone, the lid will usually flip back into place. If it doesn't, just open the eye wide with your thumb and forefinger and the cartilage pad will flip back into place.

STEP THREE: Cure dandruff-caused itching and redness. Do your eyes itch? Do the lid margins get red and scaly?

One common cause of these complaints is dandruff from either your head *or your eyebrows.* Even if you shampoo with Selsun® or with Johnson & Johnson's Baby Shampoo®, dandruff may be at fault unless you use these products (being careful not to get them in your eyes regardless of the "no tears" ads) on your eyebrows as well as your scalp.

Flakes of dandruff seem otherwise to catch in your lashes and accumulate at the lid margins where they cause itching and irritation. Some of the dandruff occasionally will get past the lashes into your eyes, where they cause pinkish inflammation and discomfort. Shampooing weekly or twice weekly *including the brows* gives prompt relief.

STEP FOUR: Use artificial tears and castor oil to fight dry eyes. As age makes your tissues lose elasticity, your lower eyelid may tend to fall away from the eyeball. Then your eyes don't close completely. The tears that should keep your cornea constantly moist leak away and can't keep up with the extra airflow. Your cornea (which has the highest concentration of pain nerves of any tissue in your body) becomes uncomfortable.

During the day, you can keep your corneas moist with artificial tears. You can obtain these at your drugstore without a prescription. At first, you can wait until your eyes become uncomfortable, then put two drops in each eye. After a while, you will know how long it takes for your corneas to get dry in different circumstances and can use the drops for prevention rather than cure. If you know that your eyes get dry every four hours in heated air, put in drops about every three hours.

At night, dryness can get to the point of causing tissue damage before it wakes you. If your lower lid gapes sufficiently to keep your eyes from closing firmly, you should apply some oil every night at bedtime. Get some castor oil and a totally clean dropper bottle. Put a small coffeemaker filter in a funnel and filter an ounce or so of oil into the dropper bottle (which may take some time). Put two drops of this superclean castor oil in each eye every night.

PRIME STRETCHER 4

Get prompt care for cataracts.

If part of the crystalline lens in your eye becomes sufficiently opaque to interfere with vision, you have a cataract. (A totally opaque lens would make your pupil look white instead of black when the light that should go through it reflects back out of your eye, but you'll probably need help for impaired vision long before there are any visible changes.)

When I started in medical practice, you had to lie still for two weeks while your eye healed after a cataract operation. Then you had to wear glasses that looked like bottle bottoms for the rest of your life.

If you remember those days, you might still be inclined to put off cataract surgery. Such a delay can cut sharply into the quality of your life for years. Why give up night driving, limit yourself to large-type books, and stop doing needlework or other fine crafts? These days, you can have a cataract removed and replaced with an implant without even staying in a hospital overnight. You may not even need glasses afterward, and if you do they won't be unduly heavy.

PRIME STRETCHER 5

Test yourself periodically for glaucoma.

Glaucoma is a disturbance in the formation and removal of the fluid within your eyeball. Usually a defect in absorbing excess fluid causes increased pressure within your eyeball. The increased pressure robs your retina and optic nerve of needed circulation. Glaucoma can cause headache or eye pain, but it more commonly does irreversible harm to your eyes without causing enough discomfort to drive you to a doctor. Its onset is usually so subtle that people don't recognize its seriousness soon enough to get proper care. That's why it remains the leading cause of blindness starting after age forty even though proper early care can almost always keep it from impairing vision.

Glaucoma appears more often in some families than in others. If any of your relatives have had this condition, you should be especially alert for it. In addition to frequent use of the two techniques I'm going to explain (which I advise for everyone), you should have a health professional check the pressure in your eyeballs at least annually with an accurate measuring device.

STEP ONE: Feel your eyeball's firmness through your eyelid. You can get some idea of the pressure within each eyeball with this technique:

1. Close your eyes gently.

2. Place the tips of both index fingers side by side against the upper portion of your eyelid, just beneath your eyebrow.

3. Press gently with the tip of your *right* forefinger, but concentrate on what you feel with your *left* one.

4. Release and repeat several times. If the pressure inside your eyeball is normal, you should feel a slight bulging of the eyeball under your left forefinger. If the pressure is elevated, the pressure of your right forefinger will drive the overhard eyeball back away from your left forefinger instead of making it bulge forward first.

5. Repeat for the other eye. Although glaucoma usually affects both eyes ultimately, it often starts in only one. In fact, you may find a difference between the two eyes easier to detect than a difference between the way they feel now and how they felt last time.

If you do this on the first of every month, you won't forget to do it. After the first few times, you'll know how your eyes ought to feel, which makes it more likely that you will note the rather subtle difference if glaucoma develops.

STEP TWO: Check the size of your blind spots. Each of your eyes has a gap in its retina where the optic nerve enters. This produces a blind spot, of which you generally remain unaware because your brain tends to fill in the gap (and because the blind spots for your two eyes don't coincide).

Hold the next page 12 inches away. Take off your glasses (if any)[1] and cover your left eye with your hand. Look at the numeral "5" in the first box with your right eye. The star should disappear. If it doesn't, turn the book one way and then the other until it does (or in rare instances try lower or higher numbers).

Now look at the 4, then the 3, and so on. Whenever the star reappears, turn the book this way and that to see if you can make the star vanish again. Follow the same routine with higher numbers. When you have found the *highest* and the *lowest* number that make the star vanish, make a dated record of your blind spot range.

Now cover your right eye and use the lower box to determine your left eye's blind spot range. Record it also.

This gives you a way of measuring the size of your blind spots. *One of the early changes caused by glaucoma is an increased blind spot.* The blind spots coincide with the gaps in your retinas where the nerve head replaces light-sensitive retinal tissue. Fluid pressure inside your eyeball spreads the optic nerve's fibers apart and enlarges the nerve head.

You should find both your right and your left blind spot range on the first of every month. The average range is five numerals (e.g., 2 to 7). If your initial range exceeds seven numerals, you should check with your eye doctor to find out whether you were just born that way (nerve fibers sometimes spread beyond the normal nerve head to make an unusually large blind spot) or have some serious condition like glaucoma. Once you have established a baseline, any change probably means glaucoma and deserves prompt care. If you see an eye specialist right away, you can probably control this condition with eye drops and avoid both loss of vision and the need for surgery.

---

[1] Some glasses bend light sideways, changing your perception of the page. Use them only if you need them to see whether the star disappears. In this instance, use the same pair each time you repeat the test, even if you have been fitted with new glasses in the meantime.

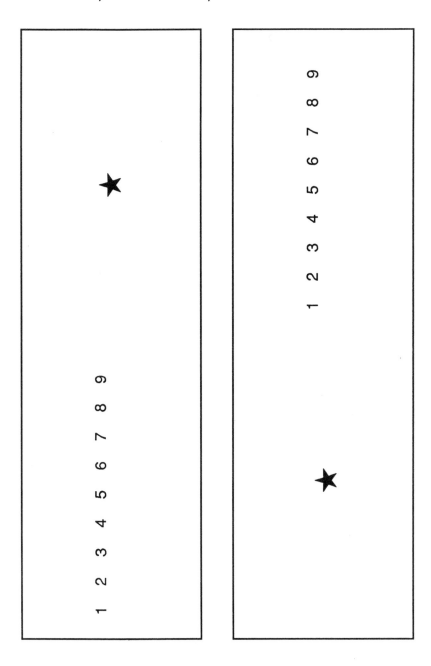

PRIME STRETCHER 6

Test yourself for macular degeneration.

The portion of your eye's retina that you use for fine vision is called the macula. One of the most common eye problems with the passing years involves this area. Tiny portions of it suddenly swell; then they lose their capacity to translate light into nerve impulses.

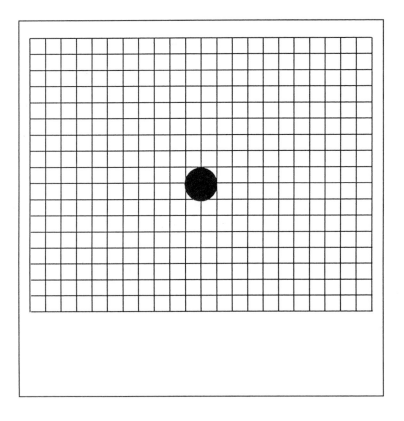

Amsler Grid used by permission of Keeler Instruments, Inc., Broomall, PA.

Unfortunately, care of this disorder needs to be both prompt and intensive to cut down vision loss. You need to spot each episode of swelling and get specialized care right away.

Test yourself frequently with the grid on page 122. Use reading glasses if necessary. Cover one eye and focus on the black dot in the middle of the grid. If any of the lines veer, waver, or look fuzzy, the patch of retina that converts that part of the image into nerve impulses probably is swollen. Check each eye frequently, and of course repeat the test immediately if you notice any blurring of a portion of print when you are reading. Prompt treatment by an eye specialist may reduce the loss of central vision that might otherwise occur.

CHAPTER 9

How to Keep Your Hearing Sharp

Loss of hearing leads to nervous breakdowns more often than loss of vision. That shows how important your hearing is to your way of life. Even the moderate hearing loss that frequently accompanies advancing age often leads to critical misunderstandings.

"I don't know why my family has turned against me,"
Lester P. told me. "They talk about me even when I'm
in the same room, so softly that I just can't hear. I can
see them with their sly looks and grins, laughing at me
because they know I'm out of it. It's just mumble, mumble,
mumble all the time."

Lester really hadn't lost his family's affection. His wife
and two children all expressed both love and concern for
him and told the same story: When they tried to include
Lester in conversations he complained that they were shout-
ing at him and taunting him for being hard of hearing.
When they didn't speak extra loudly, he complained that
they were mumbling, leaving him out, or talking about
him when they knew he couldn't hear them.

Like a lot of people, Lester felt much more strongly about
hearing aids than he did about glasses. Even young people
wear glasses, he would say. A hearing aid shows that

you're over the hill. He had never been willing to wear one, even though his family urged him to try.

By the time I saw Lester, his misinterpretations had made him paranoid. I had him get a hearing aid and helped him get used to it right away. But it still took months before he worked through the turmoil in his household that had accumulated. Ultimately, with the aid of a truly loving family, Lester got over his paranoia.

PRIME STRETCHER 1

Check yourself periodically for hearing loss.

Hearing loss can cause tremendous harm if it creeps up on you: it can damage crucial relationships, it can make you feel left out and lonely, it can hurt your community and business relationships.

You should suspect that your hearing has dulled if you find yourself frequently asking people to repeat prior statements or if you need the radio or TV louder than others have adjusted it before you can hear. Even if these things never happen, why not check your hearing occasionally? Several easy tests can show the status of your ears and let you take corrective action before misunderstandings damage your family, social, or business life.

STEP ONE: Use the fingertip friction test at least monthly. If you begin to develop a hearing loss, you will probably find yourself unable to hear high-pitched sounds first. These sounds actually are the most important for understanding speech. The sounds that distinguish one consonant from another almost all fall into the high-pitch range, and consonants do more to convey meaning than vowels: "Mpls" means Minneapolis, "ieaoi" means absolutely nothing. So a simple test for high-pitched hearing will alert you to take corrective action (which, as we'll soon see, need not involve wearing a hearing aid).

One high-pitched sound that you can produce easily comes from gently rubbing your fingertips together. Just rub your forefinger against your thumb, first near your right ear, then near your left. You should be able to hear this sound with your hand a foot or more away from your ear. If you can, repeat the test every month or so. If you can't, you can learn whether you have significant hearing loss with the whisper test.

STEP TWO: Check the severity of hearing loss with the whisper test. Whispers also fall into the high-pitch sound range. This makes the whisper a much better test sound than ordinary speech.

1. Get a helper to whisper softly a random series of numbers.

2. Stop up one ear and get your helper to stand close enough that you can hear the whisper clearly and repeat the numbers.

3. Move away from your helper until you no longer hear the numbers or no longer repeat them accurately. (Often you will think you're getting them right when your hearing actually has distorted or garbled them.)

4. Measure the distance between your helper and your open ear.

5. Repeat with the other ear.

If your hearing is perfect, you can hear a soft whisper from a distance of 15 feet. Serious misunderstanding of speech seldom occurs if you can hear a soft whisper from 5 feet or more. If the distance at which you hear a whisper gets below 5 feet, you have enough hearing loss to deserve attention.

PRIME STRETCHER 2

Check for correctable ear disorders.

Before resigning yourself to dulled hearing and learning how to combat it, you should be sure that you're stuck with it. You can cure some sources of hearing impairment yourself

and get help with others from an ear doctor (otologist or otolaryngologist).

STEP ONE: Remove ear wax. Although your ears form less
ear wax as the years go by, what forms often is dry and hard.
Although ordinary chewing causes a milking motion of the
ear canal which moves out soft wax, this often fails to move
hard, dry wax that can accumulate to block your ear canal.

If you already have such blockage, you may be able to
soften the wax and flush it out. Do not attempt any means
of home removal if you have a perforated eardrum. In this
case, you will need to get a doctor to remove the wax. Otherwise,
your drugstore has several products designed to help.
Cerumenex® and its generic imitators do a good job for most
people, but *you need to be very sure that you aren't sensitive to
them before using them.* The skin inside your ear canal is tied
very tightly to the underlying cartilage, so that any irritation
that makes the skin swell causes great misery. If you plan to
use Cerumenex®, purchase it several days in advance. Put several
drops on a Band-aid® and tape the Band-aid® to the skin of
your back between your shoulder blades. Remove it (and give
up on the idea of using the Cerumenex®) if you get any itching
or rash. Otherwise leave it in place for 24 hours. Remove the
Band-aid®, but wait another 48 hours before putting Cerumenex®
in your ear. If there is any redness, itching, or swelling at the
site, don't use this product or any other containing the same
ingredients (noted in fine print on the label). Otherwise, introduce
the Cerumenex®, following the directions on the label.

If you prove sensitive to Cerumenex®, try this home method.
Pick a dishwashing detergent that you have used often enough
to know your skin isn't sensitive to it. Put two drops in a
teaspoonful of water, lie on your side, and introduce it into
your ear. Let it soak in for 5 minutes before getting up. Repeat
every hour for 6 hours.

The water should soak into the wax sufficiently to soften
it. Now take a rubber ear or infant syringe. *Being careful not
to stop up the outlet of the ear,* direct a stream of warm water
in and toward the back wall of the canal. Repeat several times,

using warmer and warmer water (but always testing the temperature of the water with your *hand*, which hasn't had a chance to get used to the heat, before using it).

If these methods fail, get a doctor to clean out the wax for you.

After the wax has been thoroughly removed, keep it from accumulating by introducing in the ear a mixture of equal parts of white vinegar and rubbing alcohol twice a week. Lie on your right side and fill your left ear canal with the solution. Let it soak in for half a minute. Hold a sponge or towel against your ear to catch the solution as it drains out of that ear and turn on your left side. Fill your right ear with the solution and let it soak in for half a minute.

STEP TWO: Check with an ear doctor to see if hearing can be corrected. Some hearing loss comes from curable infection, fluid trapped behind the eardrum, and other easily corrected conditions. In recent years, microscope-aided and laser surgery have made it possible for otologists to restore hearing in many people previously doomed to progressive deafness. It certainly makes sense to see if your hearing can be restored before you resign yourself to merely making dulled hearing more bearable, even though the methods described next may accomplish that aim.

PRIME STRETCHER 3

*Acknowledge and combat uncorrectable
hearing loss.*

I've seen a dozen or so patients whose personal relationships have been grossly disturbed by hearing loss. Every one of them had two things in common:

- Their hearing loss wasn't complete—in some instances, not even severe. (By contrast, the totally deaf people I have known have generally developed alternative means of communication and adjusted well to their handicap.)

- They had been reluctant to admit that anything was wrong or to let their associates know that they had a problem. Some, like Lester P., wouldn't ever wear a hearing aid. Others wore aids only sporadically and complained that they could never get used to the distorted sound.

You can greatly diminish the impact of the dulled hearing (which happens almost invariably as you age) by acknowledging it.

STEP ONE: Admit to yourself that your hearing has dulled. Nobody wants to acknowledge loss of faculties, especially through aging. The mere thought makes you feel "over the hill" and bruises your ego. But you can't keep dulled hearing from doing serious harm to your personal relationships without first acknowledging its presence. You can get used to the idea of dulled hearing much more easily than you can withstand the damage it will otherwise do.

STEP TWO: Check back on vaguely heard statements and get others to cooperate in improving their audibility. Once you admit to yourself that you may not be hearing clearly, you'll find it easy to smile, apologize if necessary, and ask people to repeat anything you didn't hear. You won't need to do this as often as you think—your family and friends will soon learn what they need to do to make communications clear. If you just let foggily heard comments slide, people will never adapt their speech and behavior to your needs.

When I say "adapt their speech and behavior," I don't mean that they'll learn to shout at you. The adaptations you should encourage include these:

1. Face the person talking to you. Direct sound seems crisper than indirect or reflected sound. Also, you get some help from watching the speaker's lips. (See Step Three.)

2. Cut background noise. Even a slight hearing defect makes it hard to sort out speech from a clutter of

miscellaneous sounds. A remote control that lets you turn off the TV or radio whenever someone talks with you, for instance, can bring you into many family conversations that you would otherwise miss. If the other people involved understand that you cut the noise so you can hear them, they will accept your control (and talk to you only during commercials).

3. Come closer. Sound intensity falls off rapidly with distance.[1] Rearranging the furniture so that you tend to be closer to other people during conversations can be a help as can taking a step or two toward the other person when you ask him or her to repeat something you found indistinct.

4. Articulate distinctly. If you move closer so that people don't need to speak more loudly and ask them to talk more distinctly or crisply, they'll get through to you without ever raising their voices. (Asking people to speak more distinctly so that you can hear won't offend anyone. Telling them not to "mumble" implies a defect in their speech instead of in your hearing, and may cause resentment.)

STEP THREE: Concentrate on consonants and on the lip motions that form them. You can train yourself in two ways to distinguish consonant sounds, which are more important to understanding speech than vowel sounds. First, you can concentrate on the sounds while you listen. Second, you can simultaneously learn to recognize the mouth motions people use to form them. These two means of distinguishing consonants work very well together. One of the most common hearing errors, for instance, confuses the "p" sound with "t". Just make those two sounds right now and observe your mouth motions. You make the "p" with your lips, the "t" with your tongue. Slightly different ways of touching your upper and lower lips together make the "b," "m," and "w" sounds. You probably

---

[1] Sound is eight times as intense when you're twice as close.

make the "f" and "v" sounds by touching your lower lip to your upper teeth in slightly different ways.

Get someone to read aloud to you for a few minutes, observing both the consonant sounds and the associated lip motions. You will find that the *visual* reinforces the *auditory* perceptions and helps you to interpret speech sounds better. After learning to hear consonants more clearly by simultaneous lip watching, you'll find that you understand other people better even when you can't see their faces.

STEP FOUR: Learn whether a hearing aid will help you. If you have hearing loss, an aid might put you back into comfortable, convenient communication with the whole world. On the other hand, a hearing aid might be an expensive and frustrating disappointment. Two conditions commonly make hearing aids ineffective:

- Nerve damage. If the sound receptor nerves or their connections back into your brain have been damaged, an aid may not help you. Such damage can stem from blasting of ears by very loud noise (acoustic trauma), from bleeding into the inner ear, or from minor stroke.

- Sharp differences in hearing at adjacent pitches. While aids can be adjusted to amplify some bands of sound more than others, it is sometimes impossible to make those bands conform exactly to the frequencies at which your hearing is impaired. The resulting newly distorted sound is often harder to interpret than are the signals your brain has had years to get accustomed to.

If your hearing problem developed after exposure to gunfire, industrial noise, or other blast injury, you should have hearing tests by someone who has nothing to gain from your purchase of an aid. Even then, try to be sure that any unit you buy can be returned for at least 30 days without cost.

STEP FIVE: Train yourself to sort speech out from background noise. In a great many situations, background noise actually has much greater intensity than the sounds you are listening to. Inside most cars in traffic, for instance, motor and tire noise from your own and adjacent vehicles adds up to more sound intensity than another passenger's voice can possibly deliver.

That doesn't usually bother you because you've had a lifetime of training in sorting out speech from background noise. But a hearing aid changes the quality of sounds enough to disturb that adaptation. Even if the aid could build your perception of all sounds equally, it wouldn't match what you would hear if you moved closer to the speaker: the background noise would be amplified just as much as the talk. Moreover, an aid just can't amplify sound exactly as you hear it. Even completely normal ears hear a sound at certain frequencies as *loud* when equally intense sounds at other pitches seem *moderate* or *soft*. Dulled hearing almost always involves some frequencies more than others, so that the well-heard portions of an evenly amplified sound positively screech or boom out.

A good hearing aid has adjustments intended to let you balance amplification so that the frequencies you hear poorly become proportionately louder. This helps, but it isn't perfect. Your hearing impairment often varies a lot at almost adjacent frequencies, while the instrument necessarily has adjustment only for broad frequency bands. Also, as sound becomes louder, your perception of it involves more and more adjacent sound receptor cells. That means that an aid that matches your hearing deficit perfectly at one intensity doesn't match if the sounds become louder or fainter.

All this means that *even a perfectly fitted hearing aid distorts sounds enough that your brain's usual way of sorting out speech from background noise doesn't work as well.* Particularly if your ears have been damaged by loud noise (which often affects very narrow-frequency bands while sparing nearby bands completely), you may find that an aid works for you only one-on-one in a quiet room.

Fortunately, you can train yourself to blank out distorted background noise almost as well as you used to blank out the undistorted sort. Here's the technique:

1. Obtain a cassette tape player and separate radio. Your library almost certainly has a number of "talking books"

on cassette. If not, the Societies for the Blind usually have an assortment available. Your eye doctor's office can put you in touch with the nearest agency.

2. Start playing the talking book at moderate volume. You'll probably find that you understand better with the treble (or the upper frequencies if your set has a graphic equalizer) set a bit above the middle. This emphasizes consonant sounds, that are more important in distinguishing speech than vowels.

3. When you have adjusted the tape machine to make speech easiest to understand with no background noise, turn on the radio. Find a station that plays a kind of music you don't particularly like—you're going to learn to *ignore* it, so the less it appeals to you, the better.

4. At first, keep the radio volume quite low. Concentrate on the book, being sure that you hear and understand every word. Whenever you begin to find the concentration fatiguing, quit. You'll make more progress if you remain alert throughout each exercise.

5. Try to work one or more such sessions into each day's schedule. Gradually increase the volume of the radio until it is moderately loud. If you want to carry on even further, decrease the volume of your tape player rather than blast the neighbors with louder "background."

6. Try to get talking books read by both men and women. If there is one person, such as your spouse, whose voice you want to be sure of distinguishing, ask him or her to replace the tape machine once in a while, reading a book, magazine, or newspaper.

7. When you feel that you can comfortably sort out target sounds from equally loud background noise, start wearing your aid *and keeping it turned on except while you're asleep.* If background noise annoys you when no conversation is going on, hum softly to yourself and concentrate on your own voice rather than turn off the machine. You'll ultimately adapt to the aid much better

if your brain doesn't have to shift gears between the two different perceptual patterns (amplified and un-amplified).

PRIME STRETCHER 4

Guard your ears from blasting sound.

Of all the hearing problems, those caused wholly or partially by acoustic trauma are both hardest to cure and hardest to help with an aid. A blast of noise loud enough to damage your ears knocks out nerve cells that perceive very specific frequencies. Your body can't repair or replace those cells, so nothing can restore the hearing loss. That loss often occurs one octave above the sound itself, which means that it often strikes the very frequencies that distinguish one consonant from another. Since these sounds do more than any others to make speech intelligible, it's the most critical part of your hearing that suffers.

If your ears are being damaged by ongoing noise exposure, for example, industrial noise, you may get some warning. You will find that the radio that sounded loud enough when you parked your car on the way in doesn't sound as loud when you finish the day's work. Your ears may ring or feel full after using the chain saw or enjoying an evening's loud rock music. You can heed these warnings and avoid the intense sound, keep your distance from the source, or wear ear protecting equipment.

With sudden loud blasts, you don't get any chance to find out whether your ears are unusually sensitive. One shotgun blast can damage your ears for life. Even if your friends have been using the same guns for years without damage, your own ears might not stand the noise. Far better to use plugs or muffs every time than to find out too late that you should have done so.

Remember too that closeness greatly increases the intensity of sound. I have one patient whose ears were permanently damaged when he put his head right next to a noisy motor trying to figure out which cylinder had the piston slap.

You can get earplugs or muffs from "safety equipment dealers" listed in the Yellow Pages. Muffs will cut sound intensity by about 20 decibels.[2] Well-fitting plugs are almost as good, and the two can be combined for added protection. (Although most hearing aid dealers sell plugs made from molds of your own ear canals, the disposable ones available from safety equipment dealers work well enough for almost all applications. Most of my patients prefer them because they find cleaning off earwax from contoured plugs repugnant.)

Where acoustic trauma is involved, an ounce of prevention is critical because there is no cure.

---

[2] Every 5 decibels cuts intensity in half. A 20-decibel decrease is equivalent to being three times as far away from the source.

CHAPTER
10

Stretch Your Prime with Youthful Skin and Nails

The passing years bring several normal changes in your skin and nails. Decreased oil gland activity makes your skin drier and flakier. The lack of oil combines with loss of elasticity to form wrinkles. Hair and nails become thicker and more brittle.

Certain abnormalities also become common. Sun and wind produce cumulative effects, including cancer precursors and skin tumors. Thickened nails split or become ingrown. Impaired circulation may lead to ulcers on the lower legs or back.

Home measures help many of these conditions. Recognizing and getting early care decreases the impact of others. Appropriate measures may delay or prevent the onset of still others.

PRIME STRETCHER 1

Combat dryness, wrinkles and looseness of your skin.

Lack of skin oil shows up in several different ways. You may just notice flaking (especially if your skin is black, which makes even slight flaking look unattractively gray). Fine wrinkles usually accompany flaking in thin-skinned blonds. You may get chapped lips or hands. You may get a dull red, flaky rash on the front of your thighs and outer surface of your upper arms. Or you may have no visible changes, but feel itchy and uncomfortable after a few hours in dry heated air. You can combat all these changes.

STEP ONE: Bathe less, don't use harsh deodorant soaps, and use less soap of any type when you do bathe. You remove skin oil every time you apply soap to your skin. This can become harmful when aging skin glands slow their production of oil. Fortunately, activity of odor-producing sweat glands parallels that of oil glands, so your need for frequent baths tends to decrease as excess soap application becomes harmful. You can generally bathe somewhat less often as the years go by without becoming noticeably unclean.

Obviously, you should bathe whenever you have become dirty. But you don't need harsh deodorant soaps. A product like Dove®, Neutrogen® or Basis® gets you clean with less drying and irritation than do antiseptic or deodorant types. And bathing doesn't have to be a daily routine. If you live a sedentary life and aren't exposed to extreme heat, a shower every two or three days will probably suffice. Moreover, you don't necessarily need to soap down every inch of your body when you bathe. Soap is needed only to dissolve oily materials or skin oils that provide adhesion for grime. Perspiration residues dissolve freely in water without soap. You'll lose much less skin oil if you use a washrag (so that friction combines with the chemical action of the soap) and only scrub dirty areas and odor-producing ones (like armpits and groin). The rest of your body will soak or rinse clean without oil-loss-producing soap. And you don't need to use soap at all on your face: your skin will stay healthier if you use a soap substitute like Cetaphil®.

If your skin is dry, the best time to apply moisturizing lotions is immediately after your shower or bath. Pat your skin dry with a towel, then apply moisturizers right away. Doing this takes most of the sting out of bathing: the moisturizer replaces just about all the oil the soap has removed.

STEP TWO: Replace skin oil. Skin oil acts like an inside-out raincoat to keep moisture trapped in your skin. The outer layers of your skin are made up of myriad tiny shells of dead skin cells. Moisture plumps and softens those shells and keeps them flexible. Like a green leaf that bends when a dry one would crumble, moist skin cell shells withstand bends, creases, and friction that would make dry ones flake off.

Neither natural nor artificial oil actually soaks into your skin. A surface oil film just keeps the moisture from evaporating out of tissues beneath. Any oil will do this: costly cosmetics may have a more pleasant texture and odor than plain oils, but they don't have any specific skin-softening action. If you can afford it, you'll probably find products like Nivea Skin Oil®, Lubriderm®, Moisturel,® and Eucerin® pleasant to use. If you can't, you can get equivalent effect from petroleum jelly (Vaseline® is the best known brand), Crisco®, Wesson Oil®, or Mazola®. You'll need to let these warm to your skin for a minute or so before they spread evenly. If you carefully wipe off any excess with a dry towel, you'll keep residual oil from making a mess. Lubricate your skin after each bath, and more often if dryness persists.

STEP THREE: Moisturize facial skin. Remember that the function of oil is to trap skin moisture. You can keep your facial skin softer and more wrinkle-free by *adding* moisture before applying the oil. That was the effect of the mud packs that silent movie stars used to love: the heat made them sweat under an impermeable layer. You can get the same action by keeping a hot wet towel in contact with facial skin for two or three minutes and then immediately applying your favorite cream or lotion to trap the soaked-in moisture.

STEP FOUR: Be sure you get enough vitamins A and C. Vitamin A sustains the live cells at the base of your skin. At one time, doctors prescribed large amounts of this vitamin for various skin maladies. Then they found that high doses caused kidney stones and other health problems. If you take vitamin A separately or as part of a vitamin-mineral capsule, don't exceed 5,000 units a day. This amount will support your skin tissues adequately and do no harm. If you prefer to get vitamin A from food sources, the main sources are leafy or yellow vegetables, liver or liver products, and some fish. While butter and margarine contain considerable vitamin A, the usual serving size is too small (compared with a dish of carrots or a slice of braunschweiger) to make much difference.

Foods with 2,500 Units of Vitamin A per 100 Grams

Anchovies
Apricots
Beet greens
Braunschweiger
Broccoli
Butter
Cabbage
Carrots
Chard, Swiss
Collards
Egg yolks
Endive
Fennel
Kale
Lambs-quarters

Liver (beef, calf, chicken, or pork)
Liverwurst
Mangos
Margarine
Melon
Mustard greens
Parsley
Perch
Persimmons
Pumpkin
Spinach
Squash (acorn, butternut, Hubbard)
Sweet potato
Turnip greens

Vitamin C (ascorbic acid) helps sustain elastic tissue. Since loss of elasticity in your skin causes facial wrinkles and looseness of the skin of your neck and upper arms, you need to get enough of this vitamin to keep your skin snug and smooth. Unlike vitamin A, vitamin C does no harm in large doses. You should be sure you get at least 60 milligrams (mg.) a day, the amount in about 4 ounces of orange juice. Don't worry about getting too much. All citrus fruits or juices or tomato juice are good natural sources. Vitamin C tablets, or vitamin C as an ingredient of vitamin-mineral tablets or capsules, work just as well as natural.

STEP FIVE: Shield yourself from intense rays, like those of the sun. When I was in country practice in Iowa, farmers generally wore shirts with their blue jeans. After years of outdoor work, their faces and necks looked wrinkled and leathery. But the wrinkles stopped abruptly at the neck line. The area normally covered by a shirt generally remained almost baby-smooth for decades.

Years later, my publisher asked me to promote one of my books by going on television. A former screen star on the same program had facial skin that looked like crinkled crepe paper.

"That's what the klieg lights did," she told me as she put on heavy pancake makeup to hide her countless wrinkles from the cameras.

The main radiation bands that cause these changes fall in the ultraviolet range. The sun itself and ultraviolet lights (including those used in tanning studios) produce these rays. Window glass filters them out, and neither incandescent nor fluorescent light bulbs produce the wrinkle-forming rays.

It seems that women in old-time Dixie, who shunned the sun, wore broad-brimmed hats, and carried parasols, knew about the harmful effects of the sun. All these steps help keep your skin wrinkle free by cutting exposure to the sun's ultraviolet rays.

You also have an alternative that wasn't available to them: sun block lotion. If you must spend time in the sun, at least protect the parts you prefer to remain unwrinkled. A product with 15 rating is good enough for most people. If you are very fair-skinned, if you are using a product like Retin-A® or "mycin" family antibiotics (that increase sun sensitivity), or if you will be in the sun more than three hours (as for golf or sailing), you should use a product rated 30 or higher. Although sunscreens stay in place when you perspire (or even swim), toweling wipes them off and requires reapplication. One sign of inadequate sun block: any redness of your skin after exposure. If your skin flushes after a certain activity, use stronger sun block or apply it more often next time you do the same thing.

PRIME STRETCHER 2

*Deal with age-related changes in your hair
and nails.*

Some of the change you note in your hair and nails as the years go by comes from decreased skin oil. Although the nail plates and the hair shafts have no source of oil in themselves, skin oil from neighboring glands gets onto their surfaces. The methods described for oil preservation and replacement help maintain the quality of your hair and nails as well as smoothing your skin itself. Some additional measures also help:

STEP ONE: Massage your scalp. Scalp massage has two effects that help hair quality: it increases circulation to the oil glands, and it spreads the skin oil up along the hair shaft. To massage your scalp,

1. Close your fists about halfway. Press your fingertips into the middle portion of your scalp near the front hairline. Jiggle your hands from side to side just enough that your fingertips slide slightly back and forth along your scalp.

2. While continuing both the pressure and the motion, slide your fingertips in slow circles to cover all areas of your scalp.

3. Continue for about one minute.

4. Brush your hair straight back, pressing the brush against your scalp. Use long front-to-back strokes. Twenty strokes usually suffice to spread the newly formed oil along all of your hair shafts.

While this program will help to maintain the flexibility and fineness of your hair, it does nothing to combat baldness. Minoxidil (Upjohn's brand is Rogaine®) retards or partly reverses this condition. It is available only by prescription, so you will need to see your doctor if you are interested in using it.

Incidentally, many women who find themselves victims of falling hair have inherited the same genes that make their male relatives bald. If after the menopause you find yourself losing hair in either of the common baldness patterns—receding hairline or central patch—two different approaches might slow hair loss: you can replace the female hormones that previously protected you from the action of baldness-inducing genes or you can try Minoxidil. You'll need to see your doctor in either case, since both medications require a prescription. Since prevention works much better than cure for this condition, take action promptly when thinning hair starts if further thinning will be upsetting for you.

STEP TWO: Soak toenails before clipping them. Your toenails tend to get thicker as the years go by. They also may bow downward at their ends. These changes often make them press uncomfortably against your shoe tops and always make them hard to cut.

You can keep heavy nails from causing discomfort or becoming ingrown by using this technique to trim them:

1. Go to your drugstore and buy a large pair of straight-end nail clippers and a file or coarse emery board. (Scissors just don't work.)

2. Soak your feet in lukewarm water for 20 minutes.

3. Use the file or emery board on the top, not the end, of the heavy nails. You will find that you can thin them quite a bit by filing while they remain soft from soaking.

4. Put the lower blade of the clipper underneath one side of your big toenail. You will probably find that the clipper blade doesn't extend all the way across the nail. Just position it straight across the nail, so that you will make a cut halfway across or more. Reposition the clipper so that the lower blade extends from beneath the other edge to meet the previous cut at the center of the nail. *Do not cut the corners of the nail back beyond the margin of the overlapping skin.* If

you cut the corners of the nail back too far, you may get an ingrown toenail.

STEP THREE: Relieve ingrown toenails at their onset. If the corner of a big toenail digs into the flesh, home measures usually give temporary relief, and sometimes effect a permanent cure. If a deep spur, severe infection, or some health problem like diabetes or arteriosclerosis complicates the problem, best see your doctor right away. Otherwise, use this method to get relief:

1. If the area has abruptly become painful (the thing that usually brings it to your attention), infection is usually present. If red streaks develop up your leg or you have any fever, consider the infection "severe" and see your doctor. Otherwise, use hot soaks for 20 minutes three times a day to settle it down.

2. When hot soaks have relieved the tenderness enough to let you handle the part without pain, you want to remove the corner of the toenail that is digging into your flesh. While the nail is still soft after a soak, clean the toe with rubbing alcohol. Wash your hands thoroughly. Rest the toe against a firm surface like the top of a footstool or low table. Gently run the tip of a nail file along the surface of the nail at the side where it digs in, feeling with it for the edge of the nail. Work the tip of the file back toward the base of your nail, freeing up the nail from the overlying skin fold.

3. Using the tip of the file to lift away and protect the skin, use a clean, new single-edged razor blade to make a shallow cut in the nail. Begin as close to the side of the nail as possible just above its base, and cut toward the tip of the toe. As you near the tip, change the position of the file, placing it underneath the end of the nail to protect your skin when your cut gets to the end of the nail. Your aim is to cut off the spur of nail that is digging into your flesh, leaving a smooth incline that will push aside the skin as the nail grows out.

4. Deepen this cut until the portion of the nail that has dug into your flesh is almost free. With manicure scissors and tweezers, free up the loose portion and trim the side to make its inclined edge as smooth as possible. In the same way, remove a narrow pie-shaped wedge from the center of the nail with its base at the nail end and its point about halfway up the nail. This makes the edge of the nail more supple and improves your chance of getting the nail to grow out past the skin fold instead of digging in.

5. You can keep the advancing nail from digging in by pushing a small piece of gauze impregnated with petroleum jelly underneath it daily. Unravel a roll of 1-inch roller gauze into a wide-mouthed jar. Add about 1 ounce of unmedicated petroleum jelly (medicated jelly contains carbolic acid, which might damage raw tissue). Heat uncovered in a warm oven for 30 minutes. The melted jelly will soak into the gauze. Let it cool and keep it covered until you're ready to use it. Then cut off a small piece of the impregnated gauze and pack it under the advancing corner of the toenail with a toothpick or finishing nail. The petroleum jelly keeps the nail more yielding while the gauze helps lift its corner out of the flesh.

STEP FOUR: Relieve split fingernails. Lack of skin oil makes fingernails become brittle. Especially if you wash dishes or clothes by hand so that your nails are exposed to soapy water often, the nails may become so brittle that they split down the middle. If this happens, intact new nail has to grow all the way out from the nail bed (at its base). The nail plate itself is made up (like hair) of dead cell shells, and cannot repair itself. These techniques help:

1. Trim the split nail short with clippers, being especially careful to blunt the corners adjacent to the ends of the split. If left sharp, these tend to catch in fabrics to rip the nail plate painfully off its bed.

2. Wear gloves if you wash dishes or clothes by hand.

3. Use L'Oreal's product Mega/hard® to bridge the gap as the split nail grows out.

4. As the nail grows, it will push the original split toward the end of your finger. If the base of the nail still shows a defect, the split comes from a defect in the nail bed instead of brittleness caused by the lack of oil. Such defects may be due to growths or other conditions that your doctor can cure, so you should see him.

PRIME STRETCHER 3

Check your own skin monthly for new or altered spots.

As the years go by, your skin tends to develop patches of accumulated skin cells, skin tags, and various minor growths. Most of these do no harm, but some varieties can turn into serious tumors. By identifying and getting prompt care for the serious varieties, you can keep the necessary treatments to a minimum and avoid unsightly scars.

STEP ONE: Look at every portion of your skin.

1. Get undressed in a brightly lit room with a mirror. Use a hand mirror also, so that you can see every portion of your body. Have regular paper, tracing paper, a pencil, and a felt-tipped pen handy.

2. Draw a rough outline of the front surface of your body on one sheet of paper and one of your back surface on another sheet.

3. Search every area of your body for moles, patches of heaped-up skin cells, or growths.

4. Indicate on the outlines you have previously drawn the location of each abnormal patch of skin. Put a different number on these charts for each spot.

5. Use the felt-tipped pen to record through the tracing paper the margins of any mole or spot you don't plan to check with your doctor right away. Number these tracings to coincide with the numbers on your location charts. This will help you tell whether a spot has grown larger the next time you check.

6. Use the chart provided to determine the urgency of each abnormal patch.

Condition	Description	Danger Signals	Urgency
Mole	Brownish raised or level patch (Hair makes it *not* dangerous.)	None	+
		Location on ankle or foot or in shaving area	+
		Multicolored,* blurred margins	+++
		Increased size.	++++
Oily keratosis	Brownish scaly firm but not rock-hard patch	None	+
Actinic keratosis	Dry, scratchy-feeling surface scale; whitish	Raised edges, increasing size	+
Basal cell cancer	Raised edges, pearly color, pit or scab in center; hard texture	Bleeding, increase in size	+++
Squamous cell cancer	Raised hard red-scaly growth	Bleeding, increase in size	++++

Key: + Probably not important, but ask your doctor on your next visit.

++ May turn into a more serious condition if untreated. Don't wait more than six months before seeking care.

+++ Urgent but not life threatening. Will continue to grow until removed, so remove sooner.

++++ Life threatening. See doctor right away.

* If it would take more than one color of paint (e.g., dark brown and tan) to portray your mole, let a doctor check it right away.

STEP TWO: Keep these records, recheck your skin regularly, and get prompt care for dangerous patches. Keep these records handy for three reasons:

First, they will help you decide on the urgency of mild discomfort associated with a mole or other skin spot. Although even the most dangerous of these conditions may cause no discomfort at all, very vague complaints commonly occur. It always troubles me when a patient says that a mole or other skin spot bothers him. Usually he can't find any more specific word—it doesn't itch or burn or hurt. And because the complaint is so vague, he has often waited weeks or months before coming in. Quite often these spots prove dangerous, and they always need more extensive removal due to the extra interval of growth.

If you get such vague sensations, you can look at your records and check for even slight growth or color change. That will tip you off to the urgency of the situation and, it is hoped, eliminate unnecessary delay in getting care.

Second, your records will help you decide whether a new or growing patch needs attention. Moles, that can turn into life-threatening melanomas, deserve your keenest attention. Actinic keratoses can often be treated with lotions or creams early in their course, when less pleasant freezing, burning, or surgical removal might otherwise be required. Basal cell cancers can usually be removed in the doctor's office early in their course, but can require extensive surgery and skin grafts if neglected. If you get care as soon as your records convince you that you have a condition that could become dangerous, you will save a lot of misery and disfigurement.

Third, your records will help your doctor give you just the right treatment. Take them along on your first visit, and he'll more often make the right decisions on your behalf.

PRIME STRETCHER 4

Prevent disfiguring skin conditions.

Until doctors find new ways to treat them, skin cancers inevitably leave scars and healing ulcers leave pigmented areas. The only way to avoid these unsightly residues is to prevent the conditions that cause them.

STEP ONE: Limit sun exposure. When you repeatedly expose an area of your skin to the sun, your body takes two steps to avoid sunburn. One that you've unquestionably noticed is increased pigmentation, that makes you tan. The other is to have its cells multiply more rapidly to pile up an extra two or three layers of dead skin cells. The thicker keratin layer actually is more important than the tan in preventing sunburn (and occurs in all races). The more rapid multiplication of skin cells explains how sun exposure causes actinic keratoses and cancers, which are all disorders of your body's control of cell multiplication.

Standard Time	Daylight Time	Sun Intensity Compared with Midday
6 A.M.	7 A.M.	20%
7 A.M.	8 A.M.	40%
8 A.M.	9 A.M.	60%
9 A.M.	10 A.M.	75%
10 A.M.	11 A.M.	90%
11 A.M.	Noon	98%
Noon	1 P.M.	100%
1 P.M.	2 P.M.	98%
2 P.M.	3 P.M.	90%
3 P.M.	4 P.M.	75%
4 P.M.	5 P.M.	60%
5 P.M.	6 P.M.	40%
6 P.M.	7 P.M.	20%

While sun blocks have reduced the impact of sun exposure considerably, other forms of protection remain distinctly worthwhile. Clothing choices help: long sleeved shirts and wide brimmed hats keep most sensitive areas in the shade. Scheduling outdoor activities when sun rays are less intense also helps. The accompanying table shows the pattern of sun ray intensity on a clear day. For instance, if you do your outdoor gardening early in the morning you'll get less sun in an hour than you would get in 20 minutes at noon. If you take your walk near sunset, an hour's exposure will do less harm to your skin than 10 minutes after lunch. Note also that light cloud cover still lets a lot of ultraviolet through. Don't neglect your sun block (or leave off your hat) just because the sun isn't totally unobscured.

STEP TWO: Avoid lasting lower leg skin stains. You have probably noticed brown stains on the lower legs of many older people. These stains are caused by slow-healing sores. Blood cells leak out of inflammation-engorged vessels whenever you have a sore. Unless you take steps to improve the way your leg veins drain, those blood cells break down in your tissues. This leaves behind iron-containing hemoglobin, which then breaks down further leaving iron oxides (rust). You can take several steps to keep this from happening.

Whenever you have an injury or sore on the lower leg that will take more than a few days to heal, wrap the entire lower leg with an elastic bandage. Use the 4-inch width. Start with two turns at the base of your toes, then figure eight twice around the ankle and spiral up to just below the knee, overlapping about one-third of the width of the bandage on each turn. Keep the bandage on all day, and sleep at night with your lower leg elevated on two pillows. The pillows should be arranged to keep your lower leg level with the floor, with your knee partly bent. This improves venous circulation in your legs and helps your body carry away the leaked-out hemoglobin before it breaks down into insoluble rust.

If you have varicose veins, stay alert for congestive eczema. If you get a rash on the outer lower surface of your lower leg, use the elastic-bandage-in-daytime-and-elevated-leg-at-night technique just as if it were an open sore. Also, make an appointment with your doctor to see whether your veins need surgery or other care. Congestive eczema warns of impending ulcer, a slow-healing open sore. You will usually prevent both misery and disfigurement (ulcers almost always leave iron stains when they heal) by getting treatment for your veins.

If an open sore develops, see your doctor promptly. Better means of surface vein compression such as an application of Unna's Paste® boot (compounded of gelatin, zinc oxide, and gauze) and prescription antibiotics will speed healing and minimize lifelong iron stains.

STEP THREE: Avoid open sores produced by constant pressure on an area of skin. Your body weight resting on one small area of skin can impair circulation through that area. An open sore, called a decubitus ulcer, can result. If you have any condition that reduces your mobility for a time, take these steps:

1. Sit on an inflated rubber ring to keep your whole weight from falling on one spot.
2. When bedridden, move enough to change the part of your skin that bears your weight at least every hour. An alcohol back rub once a day also helps.

CHAPTER

―――――――――― 11 ――――――――――

Look and Feel Younger with Pain-free Feet

Nothing makes you look and feel older than hobbling around on sore feet. Whether you're suffering from corns, calluses, fallen arches or bunions, foot problems have a great impact on your life-style. They limit your activities. They make you pick shoes for comfort instead of style. They alter body mechanics, which puts strain on your knees, hips, and spine. And they just plain *hurt*.

PRIME STRETCHER 1

Trim, then eliminate, corns and calluses.

Both corns and calluses form in response to repeated pressure. Such pressure makes your skin thicken its outer protective layer of dead skin cells. When these cells pile up excessively, they do harm instead of good. A corn has a sharp peak in the middle of its inner surface that drives downward into your tissue. That's what makes it so tender. Both the outer and inner surfaces of a callus are relatively flat, but a callus still can cause uncomfortable pressure on underlying structures. Both these conditions perpetuate themselves: a corn or a callus produces extra pressure on the underlying tissue, which then causes further formation of excess horny callus or corn substance.

153

STEP ONE: Trim the corn or callus. If you have diabetes or impaired circulation to your feet, you should see a podiatrist who will usually be better equipped than your family doctor to treat these particular disorders. Otherwise, you can safely trim your own corns and calluses. Paring them down until they no longer press on the underlying tissue gives immediate comfort and helps keep them from coming back.

1. Soak your foot in lukewarm water for 20 minutes. Soaking softens the corn or callus and makes it much easier to trim.

2. Wash your hands and clean the corn or callus area and the trimming tools—a single-edged razor blade and tweezers—with rubbing alcohol.

The corn or callus isn't really part of your living tissue. It is an area of excessive piled-up dead skin cell shells, like a hair or a toenail. If you were sure that you wouldn't ever cut too deep, you wouldn't really need to worry about infection. But (at least until you become practiced in the art), you might nick your live underlying skin slightly. You'll never get deeper than a slight scrape would go, so there's no real danger of self-injury. But if you do cut a bit deep, it's nice not to have to worry about germs. If you eliminate bacteria from your hands, nearby tissues, and your tools, you can be sure that there aren't any around to take advantage of any slight break in the living part of your skin.

3. Trim from the outer edge toward the center.

You'll find it easier to handle the razor in a handle like those sold in hardware stores for scraping paint. Start with the razor blade level with the surrounding skin. Cut into the raised part of the corn or callus with the corner of the blade. Extend your cut around the circumference of the corn or callus. Work toward its center, holding the freed edges with tweezers.

At this point, you will occasionally find that an apparent callus is actually a plantar wart. A plantar wart has tiny blood vessels extending up into its folds almost to the surface. A callus has no such vessels. So the pared surface of a callus is shiny and yellowish with no bleeding points. The cut surface of a wart has numerous oozing spots.

If such bleeding occurs, you can readily control it by pressing a piece of gauze or clean cloth against the surface. Don't pare away any further. (If you want to try a home remedy, get a wart compound containing dichloracetic or trichloracetic acid at your drugstore. Carefully protect a ring of surrounding skin with petroleum jelly, and apply the acid to your wart with the end of a toothpick. Repeat twice a week. Don't expect 100 percent cure, though—the odds of total cure are about one in three. Your doctor won't bat 1,000 either, but he'll cure about twice as many as the home method.)

4. Pare several thin layers off the corn or callus.

Keep your blade parallel with the surrounding skin while paring a callus. Use the corner of the blade to pare down into a crater in the center of a corn, that extends down into your tissue like an upside-down pyramid. Quit if the tissue begins to ooze or bleed, or if you have thinned the corn or callus until it is flexible.

STEP TWO: Shift bony prominences that press on the inside of corn or callus areas. The excess pressure that makes your skin form a corn or callus almost always comes from a bony prominence. A curled toe joint can press upward and pinch your skin against your shoe to produce a corn. The head of a foot bone can press downward against the sole to produce a callus.

Both these common causes of difficulty can be relieved. Let's take the toes first. If you have corns, try this approach:

1. Stand barefooted on a smooth floor. Put a ruler between the toe with the corn and an adjacent toe. Note the height off the floor of the corn's top surface.

2. Place a lead pencil underneath your foot just behind the knobs at the front end of your outer four foot bones, extending past the outer side of your foot. Put

your weight on the foot and use the ruler to measure as done earlier. You will find that the toe has straightened somewhat, so that the corn area won't press up as firmly against your shoe top.

3. Move the pencil forward and back until you find the position that best straightens your toes. Go to a drugstore or orthopedic appliance store that sells pads to be affixed to the inside of your shoe (Dr. Scholl's® is the best known brand). Buy several thicknesses of "metatarsal bars" or "metatarsal pads." Stick the thinnest of these into a pair of comfortable shoes along the line that the tests showed most effective. Wear these shoes for two or three days; then try the next thicker pad. Whenever you feel completely used to a height, try a slightly thicker one, putting one on top of another if necessary, until you find the maximum to which you can become comfortably accustomed. Buy several sets of that height and put them in all the shoes you frequently wear.

You can get similar help with calluses on the soles of your feet. Most of these lie beneath the knobs at the front end of your foot bones. Ligaments should hold these bones in an arched configuration with the middle bones higher than those on either side of your foot. If those ligaments have stretched, the heads of the middle bones press downward against the inside of your skin, which is the commonest cause of painful calluses. You can test your foot to see whether this has happened with this technique:

1. Grasp the front part of your foot just behind the toes with both hands.

2. Press down on the bases of your third and fourth toes with both thumbs. If you can move the foot bones, your foot ligaments have stretched.

3. Observe how the knobs at the end of your foot bones move down, bowing out the front part of your sole (usually right where the callus has formed).

The knobs at the end of your foot bones act just like pebbles pressing on the inside of your skin. You will continue to form new calluses as long as this pressure persists.

The treatment I recommend aims at spreading the load now borne by the small knobs at the front of your foot bones over a broader surface back along their shafts. Take the shoes that you usually wear when spending much time on your feet to a shoemaker. Get him to put on an "anterior heel," a band of leather about an inch and a half wide affixed near the front edge of your longitudinal arch. This will bulge the sole of your shoe smoothly upward, so that the shafts of your foot bones instead of their heads carry your weight.

STEP THREE: Use pads around, not over corns and calluses, keeping the shoe from pressing against them. Pads can help to relieve discomfort further and to relieve pressure on a corn or callus when you wear shoes that haven't been modified. The pad should never be applied directly over the corn or callus, though. Use the pad to spread the pressure from your shoes to surrounding unaffected areas, not to cushion the sore spot itself.

Commercially made corn pads do this. Pads made for calluses are often too thin, or have too small a hole and too narrow a surrounding margin of felt. You can usually get much more comfort by making your own.

1. Build a temporary pad with multiple layers of moleskin adhesive. The pad doesn't have to surround your callus completely: put a strip in front and another behind it. Apply multiple layers until you can lay a pencil along the surfaces of the two strips of tape without having it touch the surface of the callus. This often suffices as a temporary measure until you get anterior heels put on your shoes or when you use infrequently worn footwear like ski boots.

2. Get a piece of 1/8-inch surgical felt and a roll of 2-inch elasticized adhesive tape from your drugstore or hospital supply store. You can make a much better pad (and use it many times instead of once) with surgical felt.

Stand barefoot on a piece of paper and trace the front part of your foot. Use this to guide you in cutting a piece of felt that extends from the base of your toes to the front of your arch and from one side of your foot to the other. Put this in place over the sole of your foot and mark the outer borders of your callus. Cut out this piece of the felt. Use the elastic tape (crossing at the top of your foot) to secure this in place. After the first use, cut off the ends of the elastic tape flush with the sides of the felt pad. Apply new elastic tape for reuse. Strip away the second layer of tape after each reuse.

STEP FOUR: Get shoes fitted properly. None of these methods will work if your shoes pinch. You need to be sure that every pair of shoes you buy really fits. Four special needs deserve attention.

1. Get the right length for your arch.

Most shoe salespeople measure your foot's total length from the heel to the tips of the toes. While you certainly need this much length, often you actually should have substantially more. Long-range foot health demands support all the way to the front of your arch. This not only helps you to avoid painful arches (discussed next) but also spreads the weight that falls on the front of your foot back along the shafts of the foot bones. That prevents the calluses that so often form under the knob at the front of your second foot bone.

People who are well into their prime (or are just getting into it) grew up during the era of X-ray shoe-fitting machines. We know now that these machines did a lot of harm. Your main foot bone, to which your big toe attaches, continues to grow far into adolescence. The amount of X ray you got in a shoe-fitting machine often proved sufficient to stop the growth of that particular bone. So many people of our generation have a mildly deformed foot. The second foot bone often extends considerably beyond the first one.

This means that the longest portion of your natural arch may extend considerably beyond the apparent ball of your foot. That's the first thing you should check: Feel for the knob at the end of your *second* foot bone—the one adjacent to your big toe's attachment. If this is beyond the ball of your foot, measure the extra length. When shopping for shoes feel for the ball of your foot. Be sure that it is not just *at* but *far enough behind the front of the shoe's arch to compensate for the extra length of the longest part of your foot's arch.*

If your longest foot bone is level with the ball of your foot, just feel for the ball of your foot and make sure it falls at the front of the sharpest-curving point on the inside edge of your shoe sole. Always check standing as well as sitting because your feet may spread half a size or more under the burden of your body's weight.

2. Check width.

Blisters, corns, and calluses form from repeated pressure, not from friction. Feel for the fit across the front of your foot, with at least part of your weight on the foot. Be sure that you have enough room for your little toe when your weight is on your foot.

3. Check the shoes for bight.

When you roll your weight up on the front of your foot at the beginning of each step, creases in the leather may pinch you. Spot this while you're still in the store, and get the salesman to put in a bight block to prevent it.

4. See whether the heel fits snugly or whether it slips up and down easily.

If you can't get shoes that fit both the front and back of your feet properly, fit the front and get the heel padded. Most good shoe stores will fit a heel cup or a butterfly-shaped felt pad into your heels at no extra charge, with one wing on each side and a narrow strip around the back. Or you can get a shoemaker to fit molded heel counters for a few dollars—well worth it for the later problems they prevent.

PRIME STRETCHER 2

Relieve painful or fallen arches.

When your feet hurt, you hurt all over. If they hurt often, you limit any activity that involves standing or walking. Pretty soon, you're living the constricted life of an oldster instead of enjoying your prime.

Your arches are more and more likely to cause discomfort as the years go by. Here's how to limit this problem:

STEP ONE: Relieve foot pain with ibuprofen. If you arrive home with painful feet, you can get moderate relief quickly by taking two tablets of ibuprofen.[1] This medicine fights inflammation. Since most foot pain stems when fatigue-produced lactic acid inflames foot muscles and joints, ibuprofen usually gives considerable relief.

STEP TWO: Take contrast baths. Most pain nerves in your feet run alongside blood vessels. By making those blood vessels swell and shrink by alternate hot and cold baths, you are massaging the site of the action. To do this, get two plastic wastebaskets, a thermos of very hot water, and some ice cubes. Fill one wastebasket with moderately hot water—105°F if you have an accurate thermometer, otherwise midway between lukewarm and as hot as you can stand it. Fill the other with cold water—50°F, or as cold as you can get it to run from the tap in any area where the pipes are buried deep enough to avoid freezes.[2] Settle yourself in front of the television or with a good book. Immerse your feet and ankles in moderately hot water for 4 minutes, then switch into cold water for 1 minute. Use the

---

[1] Ibuprofin was originally available only under its developer's brand names, Advil® and Motrin®. Generics are now available at substantially lower cost.

[2] Before I moved to Florida, I thought tap water would always get cold if you ran it long enough. But in states where the pipes never freeze, they don't bury them very deep. You can run the tap for an hour in southern Florida, and it still won't get cold.

thermos of hot water and the ice cubes to keep the temperatures right. Continue to alternate for half an hour or more. Always begin and end on hot.

(If this seems like a lot of equipment just to soak your feet, take heart: you'll find several other uses for the same stuff later in this book!)

STEP THREE: Transport tissue irritants with massage. Whenever muscles contract, they make lactic acid. If they make more of this than your circulation can carry away, it remains in the tissues and irritates them severely.

When you are young, firm ligaments support your arches. Your foot muscles don't have to work very hard. If they do need to contract, youthful circulation carries away the lactic acid almost instantly.

As you get older, several changes occur. Ligaments relax, so that the muscles on the bottom of your feet have to work constantly when you stand up or walk. Your veins don't drain away accumulated acids (see Chapter 2). After you stand or walk for any length of time, lactic acid eats at tender tissues, causing intense pain.

You can get incredible relief from foot pain by milking these acids out of your tissues and into your circulation. If you have a willing helper, use this method:

1. Lie down with your lower legs raised on two or more pillows. Your shins should be parallel with the floor. This bends your knees enough so that there's no pressure on the blood vessels behind them and lets venous blood drain downhill to your heart.

2. Have your helper dry the legs thoroughly and apply plenty of talc. If you have a lot of hair on your lower legs, use mineral oil instead of talc for lubrication, and clean it off at the end of the treatment with rubbing alcohol.

3. Ask your helper to make a ring around one of your feet at the base of your toes by overlapping the tips of his or her thumbs and forefingers. Keeping gentle

pressure on all surfaces of your foot, he or she should draw this finger-thumb ring up the length of your foot and lower leg. This milks blood and tissue fluid up toward your heart. Repeat rhythmically with gradually increasing (but always mild) pressure for 5 minutes. Taper to very gentle massage as the treatment ends. Move to the other foot and repeat.

4. If you don't have a helper, use this technique: Lie on your back with one or two pillows under your hips. Draw up your legs close to your chest so that you can reach your feet. In this position, blood and tissue fluids drain downhill to your heart and you can still massage your own feet as described.

STEP FOUR: Strengthen arch muscles. If your feet often hurt, you'll find it worthwhile to take preventive measures. Here's one simple exercise for strengthening arch muscles:

1. Pour a bag of marbles on the rug in front of your easy chair. Put a hat or shoe box nearby.

2. Pick up the marbles with your toes and put them into the hat or box.

3. Repeat daily for two weeks to build strength, then once a week to maintain it.

STEP FIVE: Consider arch supports if you have flat feet or arthritis affecting your foot joints. Most orthopedic supply stores can make molded arch supports. The good news is that these give considerable relief from many sorts of foot pain. The bad news is that the underlying muscles waste away from disuse, so that pretty soon your feet hurt whenever you do *anything* without the supports in place.

This "bad news" makes a huge difference if you play tennis or dance, or if you wear clogs or fancy pumps without room for supports. It makes almost no difference to you if you never do anything on your feet except walk or stand. So if your feet hurt the decision as to whether to use rigid supports depends entirely on your activities and interests. If it isn't going to bother you to use them all the time, they can give tremendous relief.

One compromise is possible. Check with your orthopedic supply store to see whether it can make an orthotic device that props up key arch structures with cushions strategically placed in a flexible leather insole. If you exercise the muscles by picking up marbles once or twice a week, you'll find that this kind of support affords considerable relief without perpetuating your need.

PRIME STRETCHER 3

Relieve bunion miseries.

If you're a woman between age forty and seventy, chances are you wore high heels most of your life. These made your calves look slimmer and your feet look smaller, but they also shifted most of your weight to the front part of your foot. In low heels, your heel carries 70 percent of your weight, the front of your foot 30 percent. A 2½ inch heel reverses those percentages, putting 70 percent (two and a third times as much!) on the front of your foot.

Most of this weight rests on the ends of the foot bones connecting to your big and second toes. In many instances, it stretches the ligaments between these two bone ends and lets the bone to which your big toe attaches splay out sideways. Since the tendons attaching to the toe itself remain anchored, they pull the toe into a sharp inward angle, leaving a prominent peak on the side of your foot that presses against the inside of your shoe.

Just beneath the skin at this point, you have a structure that looks like a collapsed balloon, called a bursa. This normally has just a drop or two of lubricating fluid in it. Ordinarily its walls slide painlessly on one another, allowing the skin to move slightly instead of being bound in place. When pressure from the jutting bone pinches this bursa against your shoe, it pours extra fluid into its cavity. The fluid stretches the bursa and causes pain, and also takes up space to make the pinching shoe pressure even worse.

If you understand what makes a bunion painful, you can often get enough relief with home measures to avoid surgery.

STEP ONE: Soothe inflammation with contrast baths. Flip back to Step Two of Prime Stretcher 2 for details. Use this technique once or twice a day as necessary to settle down irritation. This not only relieves pain but also gets the extra fluid in the bunion's bursa to absorb. Continue to do this at least daily until the area is no longer tender to touch. This usually takes about five days.

STEP TWO: Cut out a piece of the side of a pair of shoes where the bunion presses. If you have an old pair of low-heeled shoes, use a single-edged razor blade to cut a window over the bunion area. If you don't have a suitable pair of shoes, buy a pair of canvas tennis shoes for this purpose. Wear this pair of shoes all the time until the tenderness has subsided. At that point, the extra fluid will have been absorbed from the painful bursa, which will allow you to get back into intact shoes by using proper pads (discussed next). You will still find the cut-out shoes useful. If you wear them around the house whenever appearances aren't important, you'll make recurrent painful bunion bursa irritation less likely.

STEP THREE: When tenderness has subsided, use heel wedges and bunion pads to keep your shoes from pinching the area. You can shift part of your weight to the outer side of your foot with heel wedges. You need to wear low-heeled shoes that hold your foot firmly, like laced Oxfords. Be sure that the back of the shoe fits snugly around your heel. If it doesn't, get your shoemaker to install heel counters to make a snug fit. Then have him wedge up the inner side of the heels 3/8 inch. This shifts part of your weight to the stronger outer portion of your arch, away from the ball of your foot. It lessens pressure on the side of the shoe on the bunion area, often enough so that you don't even need bunion pads when wearing that pair of shoes.

You probably want to wear stylish shoes occasionally, and to wear out the shoes you already own. If they either fit too loosely at the heel or are otherwise unsuitable for wedging, you need to push the leather back away from your bunion. Bunion pads (Dr. Scholl's® is the best known brand) do this. Apply directly to your skin; then cover with a stocking. If the pads are too thin to keep the shoe from rubbing, put one on top of another to increase thickness.

This may make the shoes too snug. Have the dealer from whom you bought them or a shoemaker stretch leather shoes on a last to make more room; plastic usually will crack rather than stretch.

If these measures fail, ask an orthopedic surgeon to remove the bunion. If you have this operation, try to find a time when hobbling around for several weeks will be reasonably convenient. This procedure is safe, not unduly painful, and effective, but bone heals slowly. You won't be fully mobile for at least six weeks.

PRIME STRETCHER 4

Deal with heel spurs.

To date, heel spurs affect men more than women. Women probably will never catch up: before very many women became vigorously active, athletic shoes improved enough to make heel spurs less likely.

If you looked at an X ray that shows a heel spur, you would see a sharp bony protrusion extending up your Achilles tendon. You would easily understand why doctors put the cart before the horse for many years. Seeing this "spur" made them think that *it* had caused irritation and soreness. The fact is the *irritation* causes the *spur*, not vice versa. After years of wielding the chisel, doctors have finally learned that most spur operations aren't necessary and don't work. If you have pain at the back of your heel, you probably need soothing and protection from tendon-pinching shoes, not surgery.

STEP ONE: Settle down pain with whirlpool or contrast baths. A few years ago, I bought a pair of low-cut tennis shoes. This particular pair had no cut-out notch for the Achilles tendon. The upper edge of the shoe's heel rubbed slightly (but not uncomfortably) against my tissues.

I wore those shoes only twice. By then, both heels hurt. One of them got well in about a month. The other kept bothering me for a solid year, in spite of antiinflammatory drugs and even X-ray treatment (very effective against inflammation, but no longer used because of now-known long-range risks). Then I joined a new tennis club that had a whirlpool bath. The next two times I played tennis, I sat with a jet of air bubbles caressing my heel in a really hot tub (about 108°F) for 10 minutes. The heel hasn't bothered me since.

Nowadays you'll find whirlpools in a lot of public facilities. Your main problem will be finding one you can adjust to adequate heat. Many of the facilities that have a "spa" admit children. They rightly limit whirlpool temperature to 104°F. Youngsters (who have a lot of surface area per pound through which to absorb heat) can get dangerous hyperthermia from very hot tubs. If you don't get results from a lower-temperature whirlpool, you have two choices: see if the management will let you kick up the temperature temporarily at a time when no children are present, or go to a physiotherapist, whose whirlpool will always be set at the proper level for effective treatment.

If a whirlpool is unavailable, try contrast baths. Make the hot water a little hotter (108°F) and check it with an accurate thermometer to be sure you don't burn yourself. Follow up with milking massage as described for arch pain. This is a lot more work than using a whirlpool, but it is almost as effective.

STEP TWO: Check all athletic shoes for a notched upper margin at the heel. To avoid future trouble with heel spurs, check all shoes that you expect to wear during physical activities for Achilles tendon clearance. The top margin of the shoe should never extend in a straight line across your heel tendons. It should be notched out with padding at the sides to lift the leather at the extreme back of the shoe away from your tissues. Check both in normal position and when standing on your toes. When you run, your ankle flexes to that position, so you should be sure that flexing your ankle won't make the shoe rub against your Achilles tendon.

These methods almost always control heel spur pain. No matter how impressive the spur looks on X rays, give conservative measures a full try before letting a surgeon chisel it off.

CHAPTER

12

How to Stay Active in Sports, Games, and Hobbies

Sports, games, and hobbies help you to stretch your prime in three crucial ways:

- They keep you more active *physically*. Even hobbies that don't themselves involve much exertion generally require at least some walking, setting up equipment and so on.

- They keep you more alert *mentally*, especially if you take up new interests whenever the old ones begin to cloy.

- They generally involve at least some *socializing* with other people. This becomes more important when you reach the age at which your associates begin to die, become disabled, or move away. Even solitary activities like painting and bird watching generate contacts with others through the learning phase, exhibiting work and association with fellow-enthusiasts.

PRIME STRETCHER 1

Keep your present activities going through the years.

Someone once defined middle age as the time "when you've given up more vices than you have left." Perhaps one might say that old age begins when you have to give up even your more active and demanding virtues! Certainly one of the deepest concerns of aging people is that they will have to give up the pleasant activities that remain, especially the physically or mentally demanding ones. You can keep up most activities that you enjoy much longer if you follow these techniques:

STEP ONE: Reduce injury and wear and tear by working up to each new season's vigorous activities. If your children or grandchildren go out for high school football, their chances of getting injured in the first game of the season will be over twice that in any later game. Why? Because they haven't been in training long enough to get in shape.

As each season changes your own activities, you encounter the same problem. You need to get the muscles and joints you will use *next* in shape, even if you're already active. Bowling doesn't get you in shape for tennis, for instance, or vice versa.

Before each change of season, follow these suggestions:

- Identify possible problem areas. What happened when you started the next season last year? Did you get tired or winded? Did certain muscles ache afterward? Did you have to ease into a full schedule when you would rather go all out from the start?

- If next season will involve more vigorous activities (e.g., indoor badminton versus fishing), work up your general athletic capacity with walking, jogging, bicycling, or jumping rope.

- If specific muscles will be involved, build them up with isometrics. You can increase the strength of any muscle by making it work for 10 seconds or more against your body weight or other heavy resistance. For instance, here's a good way to build thigh muscles for skiing: Put a piece of adhesive tape on your mirror at about eye level. Bend your knees while you shave or put on makeup each day, keeping the reflection of the top of your head on that line.

- If back use will be involved, strengthen your *abdominal* muscles with the exercises in Chapter 19. With your rib cage above and your pelvis below as levers, abdominal muscles do more to stabilize your spine than the back muscles themselves, and they're more apt to get out of shape during your less active seasons.

STEP TWO: Avoid injuries that might otherwise interrupt your activities by doing preliminary warm-ups and stretches. Your tissues become more elastic when warm and stretched. When your tissues are elastic, strains, sprains, and torn muscles or tendons are much less likely to occur. The multiple minor injuries that play a big part in wear and tear (but that go unnoticed at the time), will also be avoided by making sure your tissues are elastic. A warm-up and stretch routine before every vigorous activity will really help you to stretch your prime.

Try this approach:

- Always warm up first. You can't stretch a muscle until it is warm. Jog in place, simultaneously swinging your arms, for 1 minute. Do a few jumping jacks. Bend your knees slightly, clasp your hands behind your head and touch your right elbow to your left knee, straighten up, then touch your left elbow to your right knee. Repeat ten times to warm up back muscles thoroughly.

- *After you've warmed up*, stand facing a fence or wall. Put both hands against this support. Reach one foot back about 2 feet with the knee straight. Bend the other knee, so that your weight stretches the backward-extended leg's calf muscles. Repeat three times. Change position to stretch muscles in the other leg.

- Stand with your feet spread apart. Keeping your knees straight, touch your right shin or ankle with your left hand. Straighten up. Touch your left shin or ankle with your right hand. Repeat three times, trying to reach farther down each time.

STEP THREE: Relieve symptoms of overuse with special baths and self-massage. Every contraction of your muscle fibers converts tissue sugars into lactic acid. The accumulation of lactic acid makes you sore, and also gradually causes the tissue damage that causes age's stiffness and weakness. Getting rid of this acid not only eases postexercise discomfort, but also preserves your prime.

You can accomplish this goal in several ways:

1. A hot shower, hot tub, or whirlpool bath increases circulation, which washes lactic acid out of the tissues.

2. Follow with muscle-milking self-massage, which moves lactic acid into and through lymph vessels. Apply mineral oil to lubricate the skin. Clench your fists. Press the surface made by the middle segments of your fingers firmly into the far end of the aching calf or thigh muscles. Maintaining heavy pressure, stroke upward past the sore area. Use similar toward-the-heart stroking for sore arm and shoulder muscles.

3. Unless you have a helper to knead acids out of your back muscles, trap a tennis ball or larger rubber ball between your back and the wall. Lean against the ball to create pressure. Bend your knees and move your body to make the trapped ball roll across sore muscles.

Kneading massage gives instant relief from trapped acid soreness, which not only makes you more comfortable, but also spares your tissues from age-creating acid assault.

STEP FOUR: Modify your grip in tennis or golf so that you can play many extra years. If you play tennis, keeping it up is one of the best ways to keep aging at bay. Tennis is adjustably vigorous, it keeps you in contact with other people, and it's fun. But you may need to modify your game a bit to maintain your capacities.

As it happens, the same techniques that help you to keep playing tennis without elbow troubles through the years also work with golf, because "tennis elbow" affects golfers too! If you play either game, a changed grip will probably stretch your years of participation.

To understand how and why a modified grip helps ward off tennis elbow, hold your racquet or club in one hand and press the frame or club head against a table leg. Note which muscles contract: those that *turn* your wrist, right? Now hold the racquet so that its handle forms a straight line with your forearm. Press the frame or club head against a table leg. The muscles that contract are those *that bend* your wrist!

Tennis elbow comes from straining the attachments of the *rotator* muscles. If you change your grip to let the wrist-*bending* muscles bear the load, you can ward off this common condition. Get a tennis racquet with a smaller grip and hold it so that its angle with your forearm is minimal. Or line up farther away from the golf ball so that the club shaft is a straightline extension of your forearms. You'll need to practice for a while before you hit the ball squarely again, but you'll still be playing when a bum elbow might otherwise have made you quit.

Get further protection against elbow strain in tennis by using a still different grip for your serve. Hold the very tip of your racquet handle with just two fingers and your thumb. This will force you to "let the racquet do the work" and keep its impact with the ball from reaching your forearm.

To get the force you need for a good serve, you'll need to use a bit more wrist. Get someone to help you learn this new motion. Stand at the service line with your helper holding both the racquet and an extra ball. Ask him or her to put the ball into your hand and then let you throw it with a high overhand motion. Then he or she should put the racquet in your hand and let you hit a ball with exactly the same motion (and the grip just described). Repeat several times until you've mastered the new service stroke.

STEP FIVE: Play tennis extra years by using "Court Shrinker Rules." When your group finds that the tennis court is getting too large to be covered easily, you can make your game less stressful and more fun by adopting "Court Shrinker Rules." For doubles, these are

1. Play on the singles court. Then you can cover your area much more easily.

2. The next two shots after the service (one by each team) cannot be volleyed. This rule has also been called the "three-bounce rule" because the service and the next two shots must bounce before you can legally strike the ball in the air. This means that all players start in the back court, not at or near the net. It helps in three ways:

   • With the server and his or her partner both playing back, nobody has to race back or across to handle a lob.

   • The person receiving the serve can return to the whole court (which is narrow enough anyway) without having to avoid a net person.

   • The first shots of any rally can be hit softly enough to be sure they'll go in without being volleyed dead. That (plus the fact that covering less court lets you get set for each shot and hit it better) makes for long, enjoyable rallies and plenty of exercise.

The Court Shrinker singles game is similar:

1. After the serve, every ball must land on the side of the *doubles* court on which the serve landed. This narrows the court enough to let aging or creaky legs cover it. If you have frequent arguments about "in" or "out" calls where there is no center line (behind the service court), extend the marking with masking tape.

2. The delayed volleying rule applies to discourage players from immediately rushing the net.

Court Shrinker Rules actually make tennis a better, more enjoyable game when covering court has become a problem. Shorter runs avoid stress, while longer rallies still provide as much or more exercise. Why not give them a try?

STEP SIX: Enjoy sports more—and longer—by setting your own goals. In sports, you can compete in a lot of ways.

- You can just try to win. That's probably the way you learned to play in the first place. A lot of people never learn any other approach—the attitude one football coach expressed when he said: "Winning isn't the main thing. It's the *only* thing!"

- You can try to reach par, or the equivalent thereof. There's a great deal of satisfaction in reaching a set goal. You need only one good golf hole to say you "shot a par," for instance. But "par" generally is the standard set for experts. It often stays so far out of reach that it is more frustrating than satisfying.

- You can set your own pars—goals that you have a reasonable chance of being able to reach. You don't need to tell anyone what you're doing—it'll sound like "sour grapes" to dedicated winners. You don't have to set your "par" strictly on score—other criteria often work better. And your "par" can change according to the circumstances. *This is the strategy I recommend.*

For instance, my wife and I play tennis in a mixed doubles group with a great range of abilities. We have an even match with some of them, which makes "winning" a reasonable goal. We haven't a prayer against a few pairs, so we pat ourselves on the back every time we win a point. Then there's a group with whom we shift into our "social" game. We know we could beat them badly, but we deliberately choose different goals. We try to get to every shot we can reach, but don't try to hit winners. Sometimes we even award ourselves "Brownie points" for every shot we hit softly to a nonmotile opponent's forehand so that he or she can hit it back.

It took me quite a while to appreciate "playing social." But now I enjoy those matches just as much as the even ones. Deliberately hitting shots that your opponent can get back keeps the points going, and long points are fun. You get just as much (or more) exercise—ten shot rallies make you run around more than points that end quickly with a hard smash. And the people you play with in this framework enjoy themselves so much that the fun gets to be catching.

STEP SEVEN: Keep sports from frustrating you by changing goals. You can enjoy most sports more as the years go by through adjusted goals. Golf gives the best examples, since "par" is such an unrealistic goal for almost everyone.

- Why not just keep track of how many "good holes" you have each round? That's my usual approach. (A "good hole" for me is a bogey or better, and a bad one can get horrible without getting me down by "ruining my score").

- Sometimes the best approach is to keep track of how many "good shots" you hit overall. Do you really need three, four, or five in a row (to get a par) before you pat yourself on the back?

- Occasionally, try a round or two without keeping track of anything. Golf gets you out in a beautiful environment, in good company. Do you need to meet any performance standard to enjoy it?

One day I found Larry C., whose golf club locker adjoined mine, slumped on the bench in front of his locker. He was holding his head in his hands, the absolute picture of dejection.

"What's wrong?" I asked him.

"Could have had my career round today," he said, shaking his head glumly. "Then I missed a 2-foot putt on eighteen!"

I started to console him. Then I thought about it. Here's a man who tied the best round he ever had in his life, and he's depressed because he didn't do better! For this he's paying thousands of dollars a year? Does that make sense?

The time wasn't ripe at that moment to tell him what I was thinking. But a little later I turned the conversation to competition against unrealistic "par" and invited Larry to play with a low-key group the next week. When he showed up, we teed off together and started down the fairway.

"Wait a minute," Larry said. "Nobody's got a score card."

"I know," one of the fellows said. "We decided not to bother this time."

"Not to bother?"

"Forget about the score. Let's just go around the course together and see if we don't have fun."

Larry shook his head and started to turn back to the clubhouse. Then he shrugged and came along with the gang.

Actually, we all played over our heads that day. I'm almost sorry I didn't keep score—not worrying about it seemed to do wonders for my game. But what made it more fun was watching Larry. By the third hole, he was more relaxed than I had ever seen him, and at the end of the round he was laughing and joshing with us all.

A few weeks later, Larry asked me to play with a group he organized.

"We keep score," he said. "But thanks to the example you guys gave me, I don't make that the whole reason for being on the course. I'm having ten times as much fun playing golf these days—maybe even getting my money's worth!"

PRIME STRETCHER 2

Reshuffle the groups you play with.

Unless you move to a new area, you'll ultimately come to the point where many of your contemporaries have either left or had to quit. Younger people may have come into the group and kept it going, but you'll find eventually that you just don't fit in. When that happens, here's what you should do.

STEP ONE: Bow out gracefully. Realizing that you don't fit in at your former competitive level can be a real kick in the teeth. To avoid this painful notion, you'll often pretend nothing has happened until the other players let you know (by word or action) that you're no longer welcome. That may hurt so deeply that you quit altogether rather than seek out a new group.

"Quitting before you get fired" makes more sense, for three reasons:

- It spares your feelings by avoiding rejection.
- It lets you find a new group without ever quitting the game.
- It keeps you on friendly terms with the old group, perhaps even letting you remain partially involved in their game.

One of the best prime-stretching people I know is Harriet V. When she was in her upper seventies, she still played tennis every week with three younger women. But their skills were improving, while hers were beginning to fade. After a while, a fifth player started showing up almost every week and rotating into the game.

"They were trying to tell me something," Harriet told me. "I could see that they had a lot better points when I was sitting out. But it really hurt to think that they wanted me to quit."

Harriet finally moved on to a different group. Fortunately, her city had a group called "Senior Tennis" that played one place or another almost every day of the week. Harriet tried it, liked it, and dropped out of her former group.

"So you don't play with the younger crowd any more?" I asked her a few months later.

"Well," she said. "At first I felt downright mad at them. But they knew they had hurt me and tried to show that it didn't mean they didn't like me. They kept calling me to sub once in a while, and I finally accepted. So I play with them every five or six weeks, and really enjoy it. I know they're just being nice to ask me, and they're hitting the ball right to me instead of trying to keep it away from me. But as long as it isn't every week, they don't seem to mind."

Harriet is getting the best of both worlds—tennis with a group that plays at her own speed and continuing contact with her former group.

STEP TWO: If you either move or feel uncomfortable in your old group, here's how to find a new one.

- Check with your community's recreation department. Perhaps there is an organization available for players of your sport in your age group.

- Check the Yellow Pages for Senior Citizen's Service Organizations or call the United Way in your county to ask about Senior Centers or special programs for seniors. If your county lacks these facilities, check your library for the Directory of Senior Centers and Clubs—National Resource, published by the National Council on the Aging, Inc., 1828 L Street N.W., Washington, D.C. 20036. Or get your congressional representative or senator (who has a copy of this report) to send you a list of nearby facilities. If none of the nearby centers has a group organized for your sport, contact the director and put a notice on the bulletin board. You'll almost certainly find others who are in the same boat.

- See if any retirement homes in your vicinity have bulletin boards or ways of contacting residents.

- Check with your local chapter of the American Association of Retired Persons. If they don't get involved with your sport, see if they'll let you post a notice, put something in the newsletter, or address a meeting.

PRIME STRETCHER 3

*Develop new activities and interests to
ward off the ruts of aging.*

If for any reason you can't keep up your former activities (or perhaps even if you can), you can certainly develop new ones. Even if they don't involve vigorous exercise, new interests help to keep you both physically and mentally active. Let's look at how you can *develop* and *maintain* such interests. Cast your eyes down the list in the chart provided to see whether anything appeals to you.

These activities involve different amounts of physical effort. Some require almost no physical expenditure so that the only exercise involved is incidental—carrying your easel into the fall woods or browsing through lumberyards looking for scraps of carvable oak, for instance. The less physical activities may not meet very much of your exercise need; you might have to continue a considerable amount of walking or the like.

Whether or not they meet physical needs, new interests still help you to avoid the ruts of aging. You can't go wrong by following Marion S.'s approach. Every year Marion takes up a new activity. Sometimes she pursues something outdoors, like watching birds. Sometimes she

Hobbies	Games	Sports	Activities
Bird watching	Bowling	Jogging	Gardening
Photography	Golf	Downhill skiing	Mowing lawn
Painting	Tennis	Cross-country skiing	Log splitting
Wood carving	Badminton	Biking	Ballroom dancing
Sculpture	Croquet	Hunting	Folk dancing
Woodwork	Bocce	Fishing	Barn dancing
Model trains	Table tennis	Boating	Ice skating
Refinishing furniture	Handball	Softball	Roller skating
Nature study	Racquetball	Shuffleboard	Cutting wood

tries something indoors, like learning to make underwear. A few of the old interests fall by the wayside; she gave up downhill skiing four years ago and took up cross country instead. But she keeps up with a surprising number of them.

Marion claims that part of the fun in her approach is deciding what to do next. Right now she's thinking about scuba diving. Maybe that's just fantasy, and she'll come down to earth later—settle for crewel embroidery or the like. But in the meanwhile, she's enjoying the idea.

Not all of Marion's interests involve physical activity, but the ones that do keep her in great shape for her age. Certainly they keep her mentally alert and in constant contact with other people, and still (as far as she is concerned) in her prime. At eighty-one, Marion still shovels her own walk, plays tennis, fixes the family meals, and keeps constantly on the move.

If you ask her for her secret, Marion will tell you that it's her enthusiasm regarding new interests.

CHAPTER
13

How to Combat Loneliness

Even the most hardened criminals hate to be put "in solitary." Total lack of association with other people can really get you down. Yet that's what circumstances might impose on you as the years go by. In our mobile society, friends and family move away and neighborhoods change. Activities that used to keep you in constant contact with others, like your vocation, child rearing, and athletic activities, taper or cease.

All this makes loneliness a great threat to continued happiness through the years. Time, mobility, and ill health will erode your stock of acquaintances and friends as the years go by. To stretch your prime, you need regular outlets for meeting new people.

PRIME STRETCHER 1

*Seek circumstances that bring you into
repeated contact with others.*

Being part of a community in which your normal activities repeatedly bring you into contact with the same people makes a huge difference in developing friendships. For instance, in planned communities where families share the same shopping, recreational, and other facilities residents have almost three times the average number of friends.[1]

You don't need to move in order to make friends through community contacts. Several other approaches will give you similar benefits.

STEP ONE: Spend your winters in a warm climate if you can afford it. You'll find it very easy to make friends in communities seasonally populated mainly by retired persons. Retired people (or people approaching retirement) have a lot in common. They have lots of free time (although less than they had expected; most retirees wonder how they ever found time to work). They don't have to break into established cliques: most of the "old timers" arrived only a year or two ago, and a steady stream of newcomers will be seeking new friends soon. And the facilities generally are designed to encourage group activities, from potluck suppers to card games or seaside strolls to tennis tourneys. These factors lead to great ease in making acquaintances and cultivating some of them into friendships.

As you grow older, there's another advantage in "wintering warm": death's fearsome toll doesn't hit you between the eyes. One spry ninety-year-old who winters in Florida explains it this way:

"My good friend up North always seems depressed. She lives in an old folks' home, and every time I see her one of her friends just got sick and died. She suffers with them through every pang and helps lay them to rest.

"In Florida we never go through that. We have a ball when we're together, but when people get seriously sick, they usually go back North. You don't even know what's happening to them until the next winter when there's someone new in their unit. You're sorry they're gone, but it doesn't hit you very hard."

---

[1] Vance Packard's *Nation of Strangers* (McKay, New York, 1972) includes an extensive study of planned communities. If you're thinking of joining one, you'll find the book both interesting and helpful.

I've seen a great many people who benefited from spending time with fellow-retirees. For instance,

---

"I'm just marking time," Jeanne L. told me, "waiting for the grave."

Jeanne had lived in the same Minnesota home for thirty years. For the last few years, both her life-style and the neighborhood had changed. All her old friends had died or moved away. The big old houses near her home had attracted young couples with lots of children, with whom she had nothing in common. Since she had also retired from nursing and had no more work-related contacts, days might pass when she saw no one she knew.

Jeanne felt miserable and blue mainly because she was lonely. Once she zeroed in on that fact, she came up with an instant answer: a good friend from former years had a mobile home in St. Petersburg, Florida, and had often suggested she give "wintering warm" a try. She spent three months there, among people in her own age group. Between weekly potluck suppers, frequent canasta games and constant contact through the use of the same laundry facilities and so on, she made a dozen new friends. When she went back North, she signed up for volunteer work in a community organization and visited a senior citizen center regularly. A year after her first visit to my office, she came in to say goodbye.

"I've sold the old mausoleum," she told me. "Got an apartment among my own kind up here, and a unit in the mobile home park down South."

What about her blue mood? It had vanished completely! Jeanne smiled a lot, positively sparkled in her interplay with other people, and reported herself happier than she had ever been.

STEP TWO: Find your community's meeting places. Almost every town has meeting places or organizations that bring mature people together. Some of these have names that might put you off, like "Senior Citizen Center" or "Association of Retired Persons." Entry age for these is fifty-five, which is much younger than most of us think when we hear the names. Others are associated with churches or synagogues, which often doesn't mean that they emphasize religious matters as you might expect.

Continuing education offers many socializing opportunities. Elder hostels offer interesting short courses in interesting localities, usually using college dormitories off season as accommodations. Many of my patients have taken these trips, often arranging later courses with former fellow-students who have become fast friends. You can find some night school courses that will appeal mainly to people in your own age group. These can bring you into contact with potential friends, particularly if chosen to reflect probable common interests, like music or art appreciation. Instruction in various arts and crafts bring you into contact with fellow students. Your local art association may give instruction and also offer local trips, live models, constructive criticism, or just plain togetherness.

If they suit your circumstances, don't neglect the singles organizations. Perhaps a few members want to play musical beds and a few others are actively seeking a long-term relationship, but a great majority come into these groups mainly for companionship and expanded horizons. Some groups, like Parents Without Partners and We Care, aim mainly at giving emotional support and opportunities for socialization. Others focus on activities: tennis (scheduled mixers on various public or private courts), skiing (both local events and group trips), travel, contract bridge, and so on.

Finally, any appropriate support group will often help you to face problems and put you in contact with potential friends. Al-Anon (for spouses of alcoholics), Post Polio Support, Ostomy Support, and groups dedicated to helping the families and victims of almost every chronic disease often prove helpful.

You'll find many of these groups and organizations listed in your phone book. The United Way can put you in touch with others. Social workers in Family Counseling Centers can often be very helpful in steering you to groups that will suit any special needs.

STEP THREE: Concentrate on groups you find most compatible. Rightly or wrongly, you're much more likely to make friends with people whose intelligence, education, and economic circumstances at least vaguely resemble your own. This isn't snobbery: it just recognizes reality. Friends don't need to share religion, ethnicity, race, or religion, but they do need to laugh at the same jokes, understand each other's references and analogies, and be able to afford similar activities.

This doesn't mean that you're a better person if you hang out at the library instead of the bowling alley, or if you eat out at Four Seasons instead of McDonald's. It just means that if you fit in one place, you won't make many friends by acting as if you belong in the other.

Spending more time at the right haunts is only the first step. Regularity counts, too. To interact often with the same people, you will probably find that a regular schedule helps. If you go to the library every Monday afternoon, for instance, you'll not only keep your books from becoming overdue, you'll also encounter the same volunteers, clerks, and (to some extent) fellow book-lovers. If you go a different day every week, most of these people won't see you often enough to recognize you as part of the community.

Even then, you won't "belong" right away. Various groups require different "probation periods" for new members. Close-knit, stable communities like small farm towns might not consider you as an insider for years. A retirement community to which all the others moved fairly recently might enfold you in a matter of weeks. In either case, you need to be seen often over a period of time before people treat you as a fellow member.

STEP FOUR: Get food and drink into the act. Meeting (or even playing) together doesn't take you very far along the acquaintanceship-friendship trail. Sitting down with a beverage afterward takes you a short step along that path. Eating a meal together before or after the event takes you a long, long way.

My wife and I go to two different mixed doubles tennis events every week, for instance. The members of one group meet in the morning, play, and leave. The other group meets at 6 P.M., with each couple bringing an "appetizer" (which can be a dessert, salad, or whatever). Twice as many people as our courts will handle always show up, with half eating and half playing at any one time. Guess which group spurs more friendships!

We also play duplicate bridge one evening a week. After playing often enough to have a nodding acquaintance with the other regulars, we started meeting one or two other couples for dinner first. Other couples join in with the core group occasionally, so that we now have a number of close friendships that started from that contact.

Even my stag tennis game has worked refreshments into the act. Perhaps once a month one or another player will show up with a cooler of beverages. We've become real friends very quickly, which is quite a change from what happens with play-and-run groups.

STEP FIVE: Invite people to your home. The studies on planned communities that I cited at the beginning of this chapter used a simple criterion to sort out "friends" from "acquaintances." You were "friends" if you had been invited into each other's homes.

At first, I thought that criterion was rather artificial. Then I began thinking about my own friends and acquaintances and found that being welcome in each other's homes was a pretty good test.

If you accept that fact, it becomes clear that *inviting people into your home* becomes a key step in improving your relationships. Once you take this step, chances are the other person will reciprocate. Then you've moved one more person from the "acquaintance" to the "friend" column.

This takes some preparation, though. You don't need to be particularly proud of your home, but you can't be ashamed of it. If you are, consider what you can do to bring at least one area up to snuff or (as second best) to have access to a party room or other spot associated with your residence. If your invitations are spontaneous, you need to keep the entry and entertainment area of your home reasonably neat. You can also seem more hospitable by keeping nibblers and beverages on hand.

PRIME STRETCHER 2

Help friendships to ripen.

You've spent a lifetime developing your approach to other people. "Win friends" techniques would be a phony substitute for the types of interplay that have become natural for you.

Friendship usually has to just happen. You can promote contact, you can create a hospitable atmosphere, you can be receptive or make mild overtures, but you can't force a friendship.

Instead of seeking ways to draw people closer, try to keep misunderstanding or inappropriate means of shielding your own tender spots from driving them away.

STEP ONE: Keep a "feelings" diary for a few weeks. All people protect innermost selves from intolerable offenses with a number of defense mechanisms. These mechanisms kick in far in advance. If your subconscious mind thinks something offensive *might* happen, it makes you either get angry or draw back.

Unless you undergo psychoanalysis (and maybe even then), you won't understand many of these mechanisms. But you can remain alert for their effect on your relationships. You can often spot and modify friendship-impairing responses.

Every night at bedtime, review what has gone on between you and other people during the day. Look especially for turn-offs, rejection and anger. By *turn-offs* I mean moments when you felt momentarily repelled by the other person. You need to focus on these because the feeling almost always proves mutual—if the other person has any emotional antenna out, he or she will know that you drew back and erected a barrier. When *you* get turned off, you also *turn off the other guy.* Unless the thing that triggered your response really makes him or her an inappropriate friend, *you* are the loser.

Henry got along fine with Pete until they started talking about fair employment laws. Pete cited a case that happened before civil rights legislation was enacted that involved the chief clerk in a college health service who made a homosexual overture to a student (out of the office). The clerk was summarily fired with loss of retirement benefits and no recommendation.

"If he had propositioned a female student," Pete said, "he wouldn't even have got a slap on the wrist."

Henry's whole body went stiff. He could barely act civilly until he left, and he made no attempt to arrange further contact. This effectively ended their friendship. Henry later told me regretfully how he had lost this friend.

"One of my sons proved to be artistic," he said, "and I got to thinking how awful it would be if he turned out to be homosexual. All a bunch of nonsense, of course; he's heterosexual as he can be, and maybe it wouldn't be the end of the world if he wasn't. But Pete's defending this guy who was maybe contaminating someone young—it just blew my mind."

Looking back, Henry could see that his own overreaction to Pete's tolerance rather than the tolerance itself was the problem. Maybe if he had figured that out sooner and apologized, he would still have Pete as a friend.

Feelings of rejection also spur harmful reactions in you, mainly because they undermine your self-confidence. But so often the other person isn't rejecting you at all! The abruptness you have noted may stem from being late to an appointment, concern about a sick relative, or having a stomachache. A thousand circumstances can make someone unwilling to spend time *right this instant* with you when he or she would actually like to know you better. If you recognize this fact, you won't take every cold shoulder to heart.

The term "anger" includes more acceptable and justified responses like resentment, annoyance, and irritation.[2] Most things make you angry because they threaten you in some way. Anger generally proves to be preventive war—an impulse to strike out when someone is getting close to a sore spot. All well and good if the assault is real and is intentional. But what if you snap at someone who admires your new shoes because you've always been sensitive about your big feet? Or give them a fishy stare when they talk about a mutual friend's divorce when they have no idea that your own marriage is going through a rocky spell?

You can't altogether undo the damage sometimes caused by incidents like these. But you can take out some of the sting with an apology or later discussion, and you can usually keep the same problems from impairing another friendship.

STEP TWO: Find other outlets for anger and resentment.
At one point in my career, I took care of a National Hockey League player who was a terror on the ice. Famous for fearlessly flinging himself at opposing players and defending his teammates with flying fists, he came on like Mr. Milquetoast as soon as he unlaced his skates.

"Most of us are like that," he told me. "We get it all out of our system with the game."

Psychologists and psychiatrists call this process "sublimation." Carrying out violent, aggressive acts gets rid of pent-up anger and resentment. The object of the violence doesn't have to have anything to do with the cause of your anger: if it's your boss who makes you angry, you can take it out on a sparring partner (if you have one available), or you can take

---

[2] See also the discussion of anger as related to impotence and frigidity in Chapter 4.

it out on another acceptable, convenient target like a golf ball or a punching bag.

It's no coincidence that many recreational activities in our society involve some physical violence—hitting or bashing (or watching someone with whom you identify hit or bash). Our one universally acknowledged sin is lack of self-control, which usually means uncontrolled anger. If you find that bitterness and resentment come between you and possible friends, find a hobby that gives you a chance to work out your anger. Maybe you can get it out of your system in a way that doesn't interfere with your relationships.

STEP THREE: Don't be too afraid of closeness. This brings us to a core truth about relationships: getting closer to other people calls for both confidence in them and confidence in yourself.

The only people who can really wound you are the ones you care about. If a stranger in the street laughs at your hat or your hairdo, you shrug and think of it as *his* problem. If your best friend does the same thing, you feel deeply hurt.

That's why you can't afford to wear your heart on your sleeve. Before you can become really close, you need to be sure that the other person won't hurt you on purpose and that you can withstand any blow he or she might deliver without really meaning it.

Smart enough, up to a point. But you need to be careful not to throw out the baby with the bath water. Close relationships do enough for you that you sometimes need to risk the exposure involved. Don't let fear of being hurt keep you away from some of life's most gratifying experiences. Wade in instead of diving if you must, but don't hang back altogether from closeness.

STEP FOUR: Let others do things for you. A touching sequence in the book and movie *The Godfather* showed an undertaker who had accepted a favor from the Mafia Don. When called upon to return the favor, he was worried: he thought he might be forced to dispose of a murdered victim's body or cover up some other serious crime. What a relief when the "favor" proved to be perfectly legal: just preparing the Don's dead son's body in such a way that his mother wouldn't see his wounds!

I think most people found this sequence touching because it symbolized a quandary they had often faced in their own lives. To some extent, you issue the other person a blank check whenever you let him or her do something for you. You know you will feel obligated to reciprocate later. You feel some concern about the other person's motives, and whether he or she might later take advantage of you.

That's why your willingness or unwillingness to accept favors shows your confidence in the other person (or the lack of it). If you find yourself hanging back from accepting favors, ask yourself why. Is self-reliance so important to you that you're keeping friends and relatives at arms' length? Don't you trust the other person not to abuse your feeling of obligation? Don't you trust *yourself* to come through when needed?

The answers to these questions can help you to draw friends (and also loved ones) closer.

STEP FIVE: Spend lazy time together. Acquaintances always have to be doing something. Friends can enjoy just being together. One of the best tests of a budding friendship thus proves to be its ability to endure companionable silences.

You can experience this only if you both arrange suitable occasions and let it happen. Leave some loosely scheduled time in your get-togethers, and don't jump into every silence with a comment or a suggestion for something to do. You'll be surprised how experiencing dull moments together contributes to closer relationships.

STEP SIX: Consider pets. Pets provide a satisfying form of companionship. A great many of my patients get a friendly welcome from a dog or cat when they walk into their homes. Some feel very attached to their pets and make them true love objects. Others enjoy having pets around without paying a great deal of attention to them.

The type of relationship you develop with a pet generally coincides with your needs. All of us like to feel needed; if that's what you want from pets, you can get it even from goldfish or guppies. Cats might meet your need for independent companionship. Dogs provide more evidence of affection and opportunities for companionable play. While none of these can completely replace human associations, they can provide worthwhile supplements.

Pets (particularly dogs) can put you in a perplexing situation: the better an animal is trained, the less spontaneous becomes his or her interplay with you. People who train animals very highly tend to treat them as demonstrations of their training skill rather than as companions or friends. If what you want from a pet is friendly response, you will have to keep your pet untrained. This can interfere with important human relationships. Spouses may not appreciate chewed slippers. Guests may not like having dogs jump up on them.

You can still enjoy the affection of an animal that has been housebroken. Going a short way farther down the training field won't really destroy spontaneity or spirit. You can make a dog easier to live with by teaching just four commands: "Heel," "Come," "Sit," and "Stay." Always word commands identically: how can a dog know that you mean exactly the same thing when you say on different occasions "Heel," "Follow me," "Come on along now," and "Behave, you X*#\@*#"? Don't be afraid to give a sharp tug on a choke collar—it won't really hurt, and your dog will still love you—but use praise and reward (both pats and treats) as well as punishment. You'll soon have a well-behaved but affectionate pet.

CHAPTER
14

Travel to Stay Young—The Easy Way!

Two of the most difficult aspects of growing older are:

- Living in the past, because neither the present nor the future has much appeal.

- Loneliness, as your friends die or move away and lack of business, school, or other contacts keep you from making new ones.

Travel staves off both of these for the following reasons:

- It gives you something to plan for and anticipate for months before you actually go.

- It gets you "out of the rut"—bringing a constant succession of new experiences.

- Going places with groups often helps you to meet new people.

- Shared joys and trials bring you closer to your travel companions, helping to make them true friends.

- Keeping up with your *present* intimates often involves travel! When you reach your fifties and sixties, your children and best friends are often scattered all over the globe.

- Today's travel enlivens tomorrow's conversation, helping you to maintain and improve various important prime-sustaining relationships.

These days, the most convenient way to travel is by air. Here's how to make that route more comfortable and safe.

PRIME STRETCHER 1

Stay at your peak during and after airplane flights.

Several simple steps help to keep you more comfortable while aloft and to avoid health problems that air travel can precipitate.

STEP ONE: Make prime-stretching air travel smoother by flooding your system with water beforehand. The upper atmosphere's air is too cold to hold much moisture. So air in a high-flying plane is 100 percent dry. Heating it to comfortable temperatures greatly increases its water-holding capacity without adding a single molecule of moisture.

Once you reach substantial altitude, every breath you take *in* has zero water content, while every breath that goes *out* carries a full load of moisture. This pulls a lot of water out of your system every hour you're aloft.

All this water comes first out of your bloodstream. Until your body replenishes it either by drinking fluids or by tapping tissue reserves (which takes several hours), your blood volume drops.

When you're young, your body can adjust to the resulting changes in your circulation. You maintain normal flow through arteries to your brain by closing down other vessels to as little as one third of their wide-open caliber. As vessels lose elasticity, you can no longer make that adjustment. Loss of blood volume cuts down blood flow to your brain, muscles, and vital organs. This results in a variety of minor to major problems, ranging from fatigue and vague uneasiness to complete disorientation.

When you're getting ready to embark on a plane, "common sense" often leads you astray in this matter. You probably refrain from drinking as much fluid as usual when you're heading for an airplane. You know that trips to the lavatory won't be very convenient aloft and try to stave off your need.

You should be doing exactly the opposite! Drink three or four extra glasses of water before you leave home, and guzzle lots at every drinking fountain you pass. Empty your bladder just before you board the plane, and the chances are you won't need to use the lavatory while flying anyway. But you'll be losing up to a pint of moisture an hour into the air while you're flying, which gets rid of a lot of extra fluid. And you need every drop!

STEP TWO: Choose beverages that add the most to body moisture while you're in the air. Cabin attendants will offer you beverages on almost every flight. But most of these beverages contribute little or nothing to your body's water balance. You should

- Avoid caffeine-containing drinks. Caffeine makes your kidneys pour out extra moisture. A cup of coffee, for instance, actually *hurts* your body's water balance—extra urine flow more than matches the coffee's fluid content. Even some of the clear-colored beverages (like Mountain Dew®) contain caffeine. Best stick to orange, tomato, or other fruit juice; 7 Up®; Squirt®; or caffeine-free Coke®.

- Ask for a bottle or can of your beverage rather than a single glass. You won't always get it, but often you will. Otherwise (unless you wait for the ice to melt), you'll wind up with about 3 ounces of fluid—a true drop in the bucket.

- Avoid alcohol. Each molecule of alcohol uses up eight molecules of water when your system uses it as fuel. Beer adds only a fraction of its volume to your body's water supply, wine barely breaks even, and stronger drinks actually *deplete* your body's water supply.

Look at what flying did to Percy S. before he learned about maintaining moisture balance:

Percy loved to visit his son in California, but he had several bad experiences during and after flights. The first time he just "felt fuzzy" and seemed a bit lost and confused when he arrived. Next time he stayed in his seat after the plane landed until the cabin attendant asked him to leave, and didn't recognize his own son, who met him at the gate. He remained confused for several hours before his brain began to function normally.

Percy's family quite rightly figured that lack of oxygen to the brain probably caused the problem. But they blamed "thin air," which wasn't quite right. The air in a "pressurized" cabin really is thinner than that at ground level, which we'll discuss later. But it isn't thin enough to cause this kind of trouble. Dehydration, loss of blood volume, and resulting lack of oxygen-carrying blood flow to the brain had been the villain.

Percy didn't like to "trot down the aisle." So he always "dried himself out" before a trip. He didn't drink a drop of anything from the moment he got up in the morning until he boarded the plane, and "went easy" on the beverages cabin attendants offered.

After I explained the water balance situation to him, Percy gave up his plan to switch to Amtrak or the bus. He still flies across the country twice a year, with no trouble at all. He just loads up with fruit juice and water on the way to the plane and drinks juice, caffeine-free beverages, or more water every time the cabin attendant offers him anything.

STEP THREE: Feel better after flights by avoiding "moisture lag." You'll also avoid a lot of the fatigue and fuzziness that people blame on "jet lag" if you keep your body's moisture level up to par.

I recall one patient who told me that jet lag really knocked him out, making him useless for at least one day after every long flight. But there was something funny about his "jet lag": it happened after any long flight, whether east-west or north-south. Since true jet lag comes from the need to readjust your body's rhythms to a different time frame, it occurs only when you go east or west and have to reset your clock. So I suspected water depletion.

Maintaining hydration virtually solved his problem. He's scheduling full days from the moment of arrival now, instead of conking out for a day at each end of every trip.

I call this "moisture lag." Avoiding it usually lets you have a more comfortable, enjoyable day at each end of every long flight — quite a reward for guzzling a few glasses of juice or water!

STEP FOUR: Dodge the vein clots of travel-related phlebitis. Avoiding dehydration also helps prevent the vein clots that sometimes follow a long journey. Remember when then-President Nixon developed that condition after flying back from overseas? I'm sure that on Air Force One he wasn't crowded into a cramped seat (the factor usually blamed for such clots). But I'll bet dehydration had sludged up his blood.

You can take these steps to keep from impeding vein flow:

1. To avoid leg vein clots, be sure that your clothing doesn't hamper circulation. Pick loose trousers or slacks, preferably of material with some elastic "give."

2. If you're tall, aisle seats give more foot room than window ones.

3. Get up and walk down the aisle and back once in a while or bounce your knees up and down with your calf muscles for a minute or so every hour. (This pumps . blood out of the underlying veins.)

STEP FIVE: Avoid problems from "thin air." Almost all the planes in which you might fly have pressurized cabins. But the air pressure still changes substantially as you go up and down. If your plane goes to 30,000 feet, the cabin will usually be pressurized to the equivalent of about 7,500 feet.

If you can climb one flight of stairs, you have enough spare oxygen-carrying capacity to remain comfortable in any pressurized cabin. The blood cells that carry oxygen around your system remain over 90 percent "fully charged" in air at pressure equivalent to 12,000 feet. Up to this point, only people with heart, lung, or blood disease so severe that they have no reserve whatever will have any problem. If you have medical need for extra oxygen, the airline will generally supply it if you make advance arrangements.

Very rarely, the cabin loses its artificial pressure. If a window blows out, for example, the extra air that has been pumped into the cabin leaks out. If that happens at heights above 12,000 feet, your oxygen-carrying blood cells can't recharge themselves fully in the resulting "thin air."

The cabin attendants always carefully explain during takeoff that "in the event of loss of cabin pressure, an oxygen mask will drop down from above your seat. Pull the tube to start the flow of oxygen, and don the mask." They don't want to scare you, so they don't mention that you'll pass out in 30 to 45 seconds unless you get the mask active and in place. But that's a critical fact to remember.

Unless you have substantial heart or lung disease, changes in the amount of oxygen in the air during flight won't cause any major problems. But pressure inside your body's air-filled cavities has to equalize with that in your surroundings. A lot of air has to move out of, then back into, the empty spaces within your ears and sinuses.

STEP SIX: Keep air pressure changes from affecting your sinuses by controlling congestion. Air has to move freely in and out of your sinuses to keep pressure changes from causing pain and irritation. You can assure such free movement in several ways.

1. Control mild nasal stuffiness before takeoff. Swollen membranes barely touching the sinus openings push aside for pressure from within during ascent. But during descent, suction develops. This pulls a plug of membrane just like a cork into the sinus opening. The pressure differential between air inside and outside the sinus increases as you descend. The resulting vacuum causes substantial pain.

2. Avoid "cold pills" that contain antihistamines, especially if you're traveling alone. Altitude greatly increases the side effects of antihistamines, such as drowsiness, dizziness, and lack of coordination. You won't get serious or lasting effects, but you could be unable to manage on your own for a time.

3. With mild congestion, take a straight decongestant pill like Sud-a-fed® or Sinaid®, or use 1/4 percent Neosynephrine Nasal Spray®.

4. Don't fly with severe congestion. You'll usually need a doctor's statement to cancel your ticket without penalty, so you can see whether any medical measures will handle the situation. Unless you can get your nasal passages fairly open, stay out of airplanes.

Sinus trouble causes a lot of discomfort while airborne, and afterward. Molly O'H., for example, generally times her visits to Florida carefully to avoid pollen from the melaleuca trees, which gives her hay fever. This isn't easy, because these allergy-irritating plants bloom four times a year. Last year Molly left too late, after she had substantial nasal congestion.

As her plane went up, Molly's forehead and cheeks hurt slightly off and on, as pressure built up in her sinuses, then relieved itself. But on the way down Molly had a lot of pain.

Since the air up north contained none of the pollen that caused Molly's congestion, a couple of decongestant pills opened up her blocked sinuses promptly and relieved her pain. If she hadn't been able to control congestion, the relative vacuum in her sinuses would ultimately have sucked fluid out of its blood vessels into the sinus cavities. Then her recovery might have taken weeks.

You can also do a lot to make your flights more comfortable and less likely to cause later disorders by helping the pressure equalization process.

STEP SEVEN: Keep altitude change from bothering your ears. A problem somewhat similar to sinus vacuum can happen in your ears. But if you know what to watch for, you can tell what's going on before you get into trouble.

- Never sleep during a plane's descent. While asleep, air pressure changes can get too far ahead of you for simple measures to give relief.

- As soon as the air pressure behind your eardrum differs from that outside it, distortion of the drum dulls its transmission of sound. Noise from the motors becomes muffled. If you are listening to the piped-in music with earphones, you'll find yourself turning up the volume.

- Heed these early warnings. Otherwise, you'll next develop a feeling of fullness in your ears. This comes from stretching of the eardrum, that feels the same whether the stretch is caused by pressure or suction.

- Equalize the pressure promptly. Otherwise one or both ears will shortly begin to hurt. And if you never correct the situation, suction will ultimately draw fluid into your ear cavity.

- Try swallowing and yawning several times. These acts involve contraction of muscles that pull open the tube from the back of your nose to your middle ear.

- If you don't hear a distinct pop in each ear, "blow out" your ears. Pinch your nose between your thumb and forefinger to block off both nostrils. Puff out your cheeks with retained air. Keeping your mouth also tightly closed, squeeze in with your cheek muscles to increase air pressure inside. You will usually hear a loud pop in each ear when air flows into it and suction-produced distortion of the drum ends. You may also hear a whistling sound as air goes through the narrow tube that connects the back of your nose with your middle ear.

- You may still be able to "blow out" your ears even after the situation gets worse. But at some point the tube from your breathing passage to your middle ear may plug up. Three of this tube's walls are firm, while the fourth is elastic. If air pressure pushes the elastic wall tightly against the firm ones, the whole tube becomes blocked.

- If you can't "blow out" your ears, take these steps as soon as possible (probably after you get off the plane, unless you have had trouble before and planned ahead to have the materials on hand):

  — Take Sudafed® or Sinaid® decongestant tablets (unless you have a condition that they might aggravate, for example, high blood pressure or heart irregularity). This should cut down any blockage from swelling of the air-passage-to-ear tube's lining.

  — If you still can't blow out your ears after the tablets take full effect (half an hour or so), get two or three pieces of bubble gum. Chew them all at the same time, so that you make giant yawninglike jaw movements. The muscles involved in this kind of chewing (not the delicate closed-mouth type) pull on the collapsed side wall of the ear's air tube and help open the passage.

  — If your ears clog up on your way into an intermediate stop, don't let that discourage you from taking the next flight. Going back to the altitude where the trouble began gives you a fresh start on handling the situation. Take your decongestant tablet, bring along your bubble gum, and be sure you keep ahead of the problem on your next descent.

  — If these measures fail, don't just tough it out. If you let nature take its course, the vacuum inside your ear will draw fluid out of blood vessels. The fluid will displace the vacuum so that your discomfort disappears. But when your body later carries away that fluid, it may leave enough scar tissue to dull hearing. A visit to your doctor, or to a walk-in clinic if you're out of town, is worthwhile.

PRIME STRETCHER 2

Control fear of flying.

You know from the numbers that it's much safer to fly than to drive. But being miles up with nothing but air supporting you can still scare the tar out of you. If you have a fear of flying, no one can talk you out of it. You can follow three different paths:

1. You can just not fly. Trains and buses take more time, but you'll probably have plenty of that. If you drive carefully, an auto trip isn't as risky as the overall "death rate per mile" indicates.

2. You can get your doctor to prescribe a tranquilizer. You'll still be just as scared the next time, so this approach is strictly temporary. If you fly only occasionally, it's one way to get through.

3. You can travel with someone with whom you have a good enough relationship to make his or her support sustain you. Maybe you'll have to hold hands during takeoffs and landings for the first twenty trips. But eventually you might be able to fly alone with hardly a qualm.

PRIME STRETCHER 3

Don't let need for prescriptions keep you from traveling.

Here's how to keep your need for prescription products from being a problem when you travel:

1. Before leaving home, call your doctor's office and ask for copies of your prescriptions, *including that for your glasses.*

2. Carry those prescriptions in your wallet, so that you have some recourse in case the piece of luggage containing your medications gets lost.

3. If you need narcotics (including codeine), sedatives, or tranquilizers, get extra copies of your prescriptions for each country you will visit. Don't carry these products across national borders.

PRIME STRETCHER 4

Control motion sickness.

You can get a variety of discomforts from motion. Mild movement can make you drowsy or fuzzy-headed. More severe motion can cause nausea, cold sweat, pallor, and general misery.

You can almost certainly avoid these problems. In a plane, *choose aisle seats.* Rapid scanning eye motions can cause motion sickness, even if you aren't being jounced around. The "sickness seats" show how this works. Planes always circle to the left, so people watching from the right side of the plane see the land moving past very rapidly. If the wing blocks off part of their view, they tend to move their eyes in rapid scanning motions. So motion sickness strikes several times as often in the seats just behind the wing on the right side of the plane as in the front aisle seats.

Sit toward the front of the plane. The tail moves more erratically in rough air.

Wherever motion has proved troublesome, on plane, ship or on winding roads, use these additional measures:

1. Keep something in your stomach. Cruise ships don't feed you six times a day just for fun. They know you won't come back if you spend the whole trip sick in your stateroom, and they've found that frequent eating helps.

2. Carry Bonine® or Dramamine® (both obtainable without a prescription). Take a tablet an hour or so before departure (or before you get to the winding mountain roads if you're going by car or bus).

3. Lean your head back, and let your (car, bus, or plane) seat partially recline. The balance organ in your inner

ear, oversensitivity of which causes most motion sickness, becomes less sensitive in this position.

4. If you have proved very sensitive to motion, ask your doctor whether a patch behind your ear would be right for you. When you apply a patch (called Trans-derm Scop®), a dribble of medication soaks through your skin constantly for three or four days. But you need a doctor's clearance before using these discs because they can aggravate a few conditions like glaucoma and interact badly with some medications.

Carl and Sharon L. came to me after a friend had invited them to cruise the Bahamas on his sailboat.

"We'd love to go," Sharon told me. "It's the kind of trip we've dreamed of for thirty years. But Carl and I are the Jack Spratts of motion sickness—I get sick on ocean swells, and he folds up on the Staten Island Ferry. I don't know where we could go that one or the other wouldn't be miserable."

I reassured them that Trans-derm Scop® would keep them comfortable, and they rather hesitantly set off. A month later, they sent me a card saying the trip had been perfect, without a qualm.

PRIME STRETCHER 5

Don't let need for shots deprive you of foreign travel.

"See America First" might be a good motto. But seeing other countries, too, helps even more in staving off old age. Foreign travel:

- Involves more planning, preparation and anticipation.
- Gets you thoroughly out of the rut, with a host of totally new experiences.
- Draws you really close to travel companions. When everyone except other members of your group is truly "foreign," both you and the people with whom you are traveling look to each other for support and friendship. Add shared experiences and you have a perfect formula for forming new alliances or solidifying old ones.

If fear of shots has kept you from going abroad, here's good news: most favorite destination countries have controlled disease so that travelers don't need a single injection. You can travel almost anywhere in North America or Europe without taking any shots, unless an unusual epidemic has struck.

When you are going to other countries, these pointers may help:

1. If you need shots, arrange for them early. You'll get less reaction from shots that are spaced out over two or three months.

2. Check *requirements* for the shots you need to assure the U.S. authorities that you won't be bringing harmful germs back into the country. This information, and the yellow International Certificate you need for recording immunizations, can be obtained at your city or county health department.

3. Cover yourself both for planned destinations and for possible side trips. I once led a group of doctors on a trip to Spain. Several missed out on a side trip to Algiers because they hadn't updated their smallpox vaccination.

4. If you need smallpox immunization, take a vitamin-mineral supplement that contains 15 milligrams (mg.) of zinc every day until the blister that will probably form at the vaccination site has healed. This will speed healing and diminish discomfort.

5. Consider taking some optional immunizations if conditions warrant. The airline you take to reach your destination keeps up with epidemics for the sake of their crews. If they suggest typhus, cholera, or yellow fever shots, you'll be wise to get them.

6. Avoid typhoid shots. They're of doubtful efficiency, tend to encourage carelessness in treating your water (discussed shortly), and cause more misery than they are worth.

7. If you're going to a developing country, ask your doctor about "immune serum globulin." This shot isn't government required, but it gives about three months' protection against hepatitis, which is a serious disease you are very apt to encounter in primitive cultures.

PRIME STRETCHER 6

Avoid problems with food and drink while traveling in a foreign country.

You can't fully experience a foreign culture without eating and drinking a few things you wouldn't consume at home. But the hazards involved in a strange cuisine don't lurk in the unusual meats or seasonings. The main risks lie in the water and in raw fruits and vegetables.

When you head off for Mexico, for example

1. Take along a plastic hip flask (from any liquor store) and water purification pills (from your drug or camping supply store).

2. Buy several packages of Lifesavers®. You'll want to either use them as a chaser to kill the taste of pill-purified water or crush them up and add them to your flask with each refill.

3. Every morning when overseas, pop a water purification pill into your flask with a pint of the local water. Water purification pills take at least 20 minutes to work.

Leave that much time before you take a drink (or brush your teeth, take your medications, and so on).

4. Refill the flask whenever it's down to one-fourth full and pop in another pill.

5. Avoid ice. It's water, too!

6. Carefully inspect the seals and cap before putting any faith in bottled water. The bottles have sometimes been refilled out of the tap.

7. Avoid any raw fruit or vegetable you can't peel on the spot.

PRIME STRETCHER 7

Don't let diarrhea spoil your trip.

If you follow this program rigidly, chances are you can travel in Mexico (or other countries with dubious food and water sanitation) without difficulty. But it's hard to avoid that occasional lump of ice in your drink or leaf of lettuce in your sandwich, so there's still some chance that you'll come down with diarrhea even if you're careful. If that happens, follow these suggestions:

1. Take Kaopectate® in large doses—several tablespoonfuls every three hours. It will blot up poisons within your bowel and speed recovery.

2. *Do not take* Lomotil® or paregoric. These remedies have been used for many years. Many of your fellow travelers will carry a supply. And these medicines do control cramps fairly well. But they more than double the duration of the attack.

3. Use Imodium® (obtainable without a prescription) according to package directions to control symptoms. If unavailable under that name (e.g., in a foreign country) ask for "loperamide HCL," which is the key ingredient and will be the same in any language.

4. Take an enema as soon as it's convenient, and repeat every four hours until diarrhea stops. Sounds like carrying coals to Newcastle, but an enema washes poisons out of your system and makes you feel better. Use a quart of water with 2 teaspoonfuls of baking soda and 1 of table salt. Run it in slowly while lying on your left side. You do not need to hold back when the urge comes to pass it, as you might have been told in the past.

5. Drink plenty of fruit juice and *purified* water as long as you have no nausea. You'll find it easier to drink small amounts very often rather than whole glassfuls at once. Fluids should be tepid rather than cold—cold drinks increase cramps.

6. Avoid solid food and milk products until the diarrhea stops. Avoid raw vegetables, bran, and high-fiber cereals for another three or four days.

7. When you start to take food, begin with heavily salted soup. Diarrhea takes a lot of salt as well as water out of your system. Most of the fatigue that follows "tourista" comes from salt depletion. Restoring salt balance will make you feel better faster.

PRIME STRETCHER 8

Make your trip more pleasant with odor control.

When you go overseas, always carry an assortment of rubber plugs and stoppers. Many foreign plumbing codes omit the odor traps to which you're accustomed. Put a stopper in the sink and tub when you first enter your hotel room. That will keep the air more wholesome and pleasant.

PRIME STRETCHER 9

Pick the right group for you when you travel.

One of the most important ways in which travel helps you to stay younger longer is by bringing you into contact with new people. You might want to travel with some kind of group; here are a few elements to look for in making arrangements:

- Common interests. People who share your own involvements make good traveling companions. Consider taking an "elder hostel" course or signing up for a "theater" or "garden" trip. You can go with a group from a club or organization to which you now belong.
- Proper balance of sightseeing and free time. Lots of "attractions" mean lots of regimentation and lots of physical demand. How much of both will suit you and any traveling companion?
- Affordability. You'll enjoy yourself more if you have cash for extras and souvenirs. Don't take the "all expenses included" label seriously.

If you aren't seeking new friends, and if both you and your companions are experienced travelers, consider going independently, perhaps even without the assistance of travel agents. Many of the best foreign facilities I've enjoyed aren't available through agents, including the government-run paradors of Spain and a house-and-car trade with an English family (arranged through a club).

Have fun, make friends, and build memories with travel!

CHAPTER

15

Sleep Well, Live Well

You feel better and function better if you get all the sleep you need. I can't tell you exactly how many hours you need to spend in bed at night to feel in your prime. You need less and less as the years go by, but different people have very different requirements. The methods in this section will help you to meet your needs efficiently, though, whatever those needs may be.

PRIME STRETCHER 1

*Dodge the sleeplessness-anxiety-more
sleeplessness vicious circle.*

What do you do when you can't get to sleep?

Lots of people lie there and say to themselves: "Another bad night! I won't be worth anything in the morning." The more they fret, the worse it gets, and the prophecy of not being worth anything in the morning soon fulfills itself.

STEP ONE: Stay calm and just rest. Scientific studies show that your body actually burns more energy during sleep than it does during rest. Once you get past a very minimum amount of sleep, just resting quietly does as much as sleep to recharge your batteries.

Of course, tossing and turning or stewing about your insomnia don't qualify as rest, so your first weapon against sleeplessness is unconcern. If you can shrug your shoulders and

213

relax, you'll be surprised at how thoroughly rested you will feel in the morning.

STEP TWO: Limit stimulant intake. My first medical practice was in an Iowa farm town. Community life revolved around coffee, which was served at every gathering. The doctors' lounge and every nursing station of every hospital featured coffee. Farm folk kept a pot of water boiling on the corncob-fired stove and poured it into the top of a drip coffee maker whenever they heard the gravel scrunch, without even looking to see who had arrived. After one busy day, I counted up the cups I had consumed and reached twenty-three. But I still slept like a baby.

A few years later, I had to set a six-cup limit. In my forties, even those needed to be half decaffeinated, and today (at seventy) any caffeine after noon (and more than a cup or so before) affects my sleep.

Many of my patients have had the same experience. Stimulants affect you much more profoundly as the years go by. This effect becomes noticeable in your thirties or forties and gets greater every year thereafter.

The stimulant you most often encounter is caffeine, which is present not only in coffee and tea but also in cola drinks, Mountain Dew® and several other soft drinks. Two chemical cousins of caffeine, theophylline and theobromine, also pervade our culture. About half the stimulant in tea is caffeine, the other half being theophylline. Thus even decaffeinated tea has considerable stimulant action. Cocoa contains theobromine. Many people need to avoid cocoa products like chocolate bars and chocolate syrup in the evening to sleep well.

STEP THREE: See if sugars are a stimulant for you. When you consume sugars and starches, your system converts them into glucose and then stores any excess as glycogen. When your system needs extra glucose, it makes it from the stored glycogen. The speed at which you store and retrieve glucose varies considerably. If your system keeps the level of glucose almost constant, you are a slow metabolizer whose system uses sugars gradually over a period of time. Sugars and starches probably don't give you a lift, and also don't interfere with your sleep. If your system lets your glucose level swing up when you consume sugars and drop down later, you are a fast metabolizer. Sugars and starches may give you a quick burst of energy. Or you may get effects mainly from the later drop in blood sugar, such as headaches, dizziness, or fatigue that vanishes almost instantly when you suck a mint or drink orange juice or nondiet soda.

If you have noticed either of these effects—a burst of energy from sugars or complaints readily relieved by sugars when you haven't recently eaten—you should avoid food for at least two hours before bedtime. You'll probably find that this will help you to get to sleep more promptly. As a fast metabolizer, you may then find that you tend to awaken in the middle of the night when your blood sugar has dropped below normal. Often sucking a Swedish mint or taking a few swallows of orange juice will help you get back to sleep more quickly. (If you have other complaints from wide blood sugar swings, you may be able to control them and also improve your sleep pattern with the measures suggested for hypoglycemic headaches in Chapter 17.)

STEP FOUR: Prepare a quiet activity for sleepless intervals. Sometimes you just can't lie there and rest without feeling annoyed, or your sleep needs simply differ from those of the rest of the household so that you're wide awake at times when normal activity would disturb others.

My patients have found various solutions to this problem. Some get "books on tape" from the library and listen to them through earphones. Music through earphones offers another choice. Modern orthophonic earphones give amazing sound reproduction, making their use no real sacrifice in sound quality. If light won't bother the other people, a number of quiet activities become possible: reading, knitting, or doing crossword puzzles, for instance. Usually an hour or less of quiet activity gets you ready to give bed another try, if it isn't yet time to get up.

PRIME STRETCHER 2

*Decrease your sleep need by learning
progressive muscular relaxation.*

You can cut your need for sleep considerably by various techniques of relaxation. These techniques actually reduce your body's
fuel use well below that during sleep. A 20-minute relaxation
interval usually cuts your sleep need about 1 hour. Briefer
relaxation intervals that you can fit into odd (otherwise wasted)
moments work almost as well. These ways of *replacing* sleep
often keep your mind and body fully efficient when means of
improving its quality are ineffective.

**STEP ONE: Learn to relax your various muscle groups under
ideal conditions.** No one knows how to relax muscles without
spending some time and effort learning the art. People (including
doctors) who tell you to "just relax" don't understand the situation
at all. But you *can* learn to loosen up tense muscles if you
spend some time and effort on the following technique. You'll
need to spend about half an hour a day for three or four
weeks learning to use it, but the results (both in control of
sleeplessness and in control of tension itself) more than justify
the effort.

1. At first, you will need to remove all physical and mental
   distractions.

   - Lie down in a quiet, darkened room.
   - Support your lower legs and arms level with the
     ground on pillows.
   - Close your eyes.

2. Now use the fact that you already know how to *contract*
   muscles to learn to *relax* them.

   - Hold your neck a little bit stiff, then moderately stiff,
     then very stiff, then as stiff as you can make it.
   - Now move back down that scale to very stiff, then
     to moderately stiff, then to a little stiff, then to normal.

3. Now *go one step farther*, relaxing the muscles beyond their normal state.

4. Practice this several times, until you have the feel of loosening up a muscle beyond its normal "resting" state.

5. Now try to do the same with the muscles of your right shoulder, then your right upper arm, lower arm, then hand.

6. Continue around your whole body, relaxing muscle groups in your right leg, left leg, left arm, back, abdomen, face, and scalp.

7. When you have relaxed every muscle group in your body, take time out for three deep breaths. Then start around again, relaxing each muscle group a bit further than you left it last time around.

8. Continue for about 20 minutes, by which time you should feel thoroughly relaxed.

If you follow this method at least once a day for three weeks, you will find yourself more and more able to relax muscles at will. Your sleep need will decrease substantially, and you may find that this relaxation technique helps you relieve anxieties at night.

You can benefit further from the progressive muscular relaxation method by using it to break the buildup of tension during the day and to make use of otherwise-wasted moments.

STEP TWO: Work many "refresher slouch" intervals into your day. If you have trouble getting to sleep, rather than waking early or in the middle of the night, tensions that build up during the day are often the cause of the problem. The effect of tension on nerves and muscles is closely linked. If you relieve muscle tension, you also ease the tension or anxiety you feel and decrease the sleep-impairing impact of those emotions.

Once you have learned under ideal circumstances to control muscle tension consciously with progressive muscular relaxation, you can relax your muscles without going through the whole routine. Whenever tension begins to build up, spend 2 or 3 minutes on a "refresher slouch," following these directions:

1. Sit in a straight chair with both feet on the ground.
2. Put both hands on your knees.
3. Let your head slump forward onto your chest.
4. Now relax each of your body parts in succession, going "around," then "up." Relax:
   - your right shoulder, upper arm, forearm, hand
   - your right thigh, lower leg, and foot
   - your left thigh, lower leg, and foot
   - your left shoulder, upper arm, forearm, hand
   - your abdominal muscles
   - your lower back
   - your upper back
   - your neck
   - your face and forehead
   - your scalp
5. Take a deep breath and start another go-round. Continue for about 2 minutes.

PRIME STRETCHER 3

Wean yourself away from sedatives and tranquilizers.

Every sleeping pill on the market has one thing in common: after three weeks or less of regular use, the dose that originally put you to sleep ceases to work. The change in your system that makes the drug ineffective also makes you dependent on it: if you quit, you'll endure a few worse than usual sleepless nights before you get back to your usual status (which still isn't perfect or you wouldn't have started the pills in the first place).

If your sleeplessness hasn't been too bad and the length of time on sedatives fairly short, you may be able to quit cold turkey. Otherwise, you'll find it worthwhile to spend 45 minutes before bedtime on this procedure:

STEP ONE: Take a tranquilizing tub bath at bedtime.

1. Set a timer for 45 minutes, in case you fall asleep during this very relaxing routine.

2. Fill your tub with tepid water, 96°F to 98°F.

3. Tie a washrag or length of gauze to the faucet, so that the water runs down it instead of splashing into the tub.

4. Get in and make yourself comfortable, using a rolled towel under the back of your neck as a pillow.

5. Adjust the taps so that a slow stream of water at that same temperature constantly enters the tub (and leaves through the overflow drain).

6. Lie quietly in the tub, stirring only to avoid stiffness or discomfort, for 45 minutes. You will find that after the first half hour, your body gradually relaxes completely.

Use this method of relaxing before you go to bed for at least a week after you stop taking sleeping pills if you have been on them for some time.

STEP TWO: Get away from tranquilizers with the aid of relaxation techniques. The progressive muscular relaxation and refresher slouch techniques discussed earlier in this chapter can help you wean yourself away from tranquilizers. If you have been taking these for some time, follow the three-week learning period for progressive muscular relaxation before you try to taper your pills. Continue that whole technique, including the darkened room and half-hour time span, at least once a day while you taper and quit your tranquilizers.

When you have thoroughly mastered the relaxation techniques, you will find that you can use almost every otherwise-wasted moment throughout your day to keep tension from building up. While waiting for stop lights when driving, while on "hold" on the telephone, during commercials when watching TV—dozens of times a day you can take a moment to see whether any muscles have tensed up and to relax them. You'll find that doing so very effectively keeps anxiety and tension from building up.

PRIME STRETCHER 4

Identify and get care for serious sleep disturbances.

If you frequently wake up very early in the morning and can't get back to sleep, you may be sliding into depression.

STEP ONE: Get a doctor's help if the evidence suggests depression. If two or more of the following signs appear, a visit to your doctor will certainly be worthwhile:

1. A blue mood, especially when you first wake up in the morning
2. Constipation
3. Involuntary weight loss
4. Loss of interest in or capacity for sex

These signs point to the type of depression that stems from correctable chemical changes in the brain. When one of your brain cells seeks to stimulate another, it squirts out a chemical called dopamine. An eraser enzyme called dopaminase gets rid of the dopamine after it has done its job. If your system forms too little dopaminase, the target nerve cells keep firing and firing until they exhaust themselves. Blue moods and the other changes described above result.

Although you can almost always find some recent reversal or misstep to blame your blue mood on, depression with these signs almost always stems from physical rather than situational difficulties and ultimately responds well to treatment with appropriate medicines. Response may be slow. The medicines that work best in the long run often take three to four weeks to assert themselves. But the effects are worth waiting for: one or another antidepressant almost always can bring back a cheerful outlook, a good night's sleep, and reversal of the physical difficulties attributable to the disorder.

STEP TWO: Get someone to observe your breathing patterns while you are sound asleep. If you often wake up not feeling rested, you may be sleeping poorly because of sleep apnea (Greek for "no breathing"). Victims of this condition intermittently stop breathing for 45 seconds or more when they get into the deeper planes of sleep. The need for air partially rouses them, and they start breathing again without waking up all the way. But the apnea not only interferes with sound sleep but also can weaken your heart and circulation.

Certain other characteristics suggest that you might have this condition:

- Loud snoring. The most common kind of sleep apnea occurs when tissues of the nasopharynx block your breathing passage whenever the surrounding muscles relax. When partially relaxed these tissues will vibrate in the airstream, so victims of sleep apnea often (but not always) snore heavily.

- Poor sleep after consuming alcohol. Alcohol tends to relax muscles in the part of the breathing passage concerned, which adds to the already dangerous laxity of sleep apnea.

- Bad results from sleeping pills. The muscle-relaxing effect of sleeping pills often aggravates sleep apnea, more than overcoming any benefit the tablets might (at least temporarily) have.

- Erratic blood pressure readings. Although most of the patients I have found to have sleep apnea were in their forties or fifties, one was only fourteen. The morning after he had a bad night his blood pressure read 214/112 (both numbers about twice what they should be). Later the same day his readings were normal.

While many other things can cause wildly fluctuating blood pressure readings, sleep apnea is one of the easiest to correct (and definitely the easiest to detect without expensive or uncomfortable tests).

If any of these signs makes you suspect that you might have sleep apnea, the simplest test is to have someone watch you sleep. It may help to have on hand a piece of very light cloth like a veil with which to detect air currents.

1. Before going to sleep, pinch your nose and close your mouth to cut off airflow completely and try to breathe heavily against the obstruction. Have your helper observe how your chest and abdomen move. When breathing is obstructed, trying to inflate your chest sucks in your abdomen. It is important that your helper be able to recognize this pattern and distinguish it from normal respiration.

2. Next, go to sleep with your helper watching. You will have to reach the deeper sleep planes before the condition shows up, so your helper should plan to watch you for at least three hours. If an apneic episode occurs, your normal breathing rhythm will be interrupted by a pause. This may be followed by intense reciprocal chest and abdomen movements as you struggle for air against the closed-off pharynx. If your helper is in doubt about whether air is flowing in and out, placing the thin veil over your nose and mouth should settle the issue.

3. While some brief interruptions in breathing rhythm occur normally during sleep, these seldom last more than 30 seconds. If the interruption lasts more than 45 seconds, sleep apnea is definitely present. If this condition has been plaguing you, several such episodes (from three or four to fifteen or twenty) may occur during an hour of sound sleep.

If your home test seems suspicious but not certain, a sleep disorder center can do more precise tests, recording airflow with a sensitive instrument and determining sleep plane with brain waves. Correction usually calls for some kind of surgery by an ear, nose, and throat specialist (otolaryngologist). If you actually have sleep apnea, you'll be amazed at how much better you'll feel after getting it corrected. Both your sleep pattern and your circulation will tremendously improve. One of my patients remarked, "I feel twenty years younger!"

CHAPTER
16

Keep Your Memory Sharp with Four Simple Techniques

You've heard jokes like the one about the three elderly golfers who couldn't keep track of their balls because of poor vision. The club pro suggested that they play with a keen-eyed oldster, who carefully watched each shot and assured the others that he knew exactly where each ball had come to rest. But when they walked down the fairway together and asked where the balls were, the keen-eyed oldster answered: "Darn if I can remember."

Perhaps amusing as a joke, but no fun at all when something similar happens to *you*. Even the best preserved prime stretchers find themselves groping for a familiar name or blanking out on a well-known fact occasionally.

PRIME STRETCHER 1

Don't be unduly concerned about an occasional memory gap.

With all the talk about Alzheimer's, it's very easy to find yourself fretting about any and every memory gap. At least two varieties of memory failure have no serious significance. Memory gaps that fit into these categories shouldn't disturb you:

- Full computer slot problems. Everybody remembers the license plate number of his or her first car. By your tenth it isn't that easy. Likewise with telephone numbers: not only are they longer now than they were when you were young, but you've memorized a hundred or more without ever erasing one (your brain doesn't have a "delete" button). Remembering where you put your glasses or parked the car fall into the same category: you've done the same thing so often that your brain no longer has a convenient empty pigeonhole for new facts. Don't be worried if you're finding it harder to recollect this kind of thing. Everyone finds it harder and harder to replace old facts with quite similar new ones.

- Momentary blocks. If you're over forty, chances are you occasionally find yourself unable to recall some very familiar fact, like a close friend's name or your daughter's street address. You grope for it futilely, then a few minutes later it just pops back into your mind.

Aggravating as these episodes may be, they don't mean that you have Alzheimer's or any other condition that is likely to wipe out your mental functions. You can take several actions, which we'll discuss in the rest of this section, to unburden and improve your memory. But don't let a few overloaded circuits or temporary blocks make you anxious or depressed. Undue concern about these normal results of aging just makes them more aggravating and worse.

PRIME STRETCHER 2

Unburden your memory with routines and records.

Memory gaps will plague you much less if you organize your routines and records to decrease your memory need. If you haven't already taken them, these simple steps will greatly unburden your memory:

STEP ONE: Establish shopping routines. Shopping involves a lot of memory: what you need, where to find it, where you left the car, and so on. You can take a lot of strain off your memory by establishing specific routines. If you haven't already adopted them, use the following techniques.

1. Don't just write down things you'll need the next time you shop; write them down in aisle-organized categories. Whenever I shopped for groceries, I used to need to check over the list before getting into the checkout line. I almost always found that I had forgotten an item and had to go back for it. Finally I wrote down the main categories and assigned them numbers according to my usual route through the store. I bought a clipboard for my grocery list and wrote the numbers along the edge with a felt-tipped pen, spaced out according to how many items I usually need in each group. By clipping a clean lined sheet to the board and assembling my list already sorted into categories, I not only shop more efficiently, I also avoid being reminded once a week that my memory isn't what it once was.

Sample Shopping Route

1. Dairy
2. Canned meats, fish, fruits, and vegetables
3. Toiletries
4. Soup, seasonings, pasta
5. Coffee, jam, cake mixes, cereals
6. Soaps and cleansers
7. Beverages
8. Meats
9. Fresh produce
10. Bread and bakery
11. Reading matter
12. Frozen products

---

2. Pick the best day (or days) and the best time for shopping and stick to that schedule.

3. Before setting out for the store, check your calendar to see how many meals you will prepare before your

next shopping trip and figure out what you will need for each of them. Especially if you live alone, this will serve two purposes: it will organize your shopping and give you an overview of your eating patterns.

4. Keep a separate list for things you need from other stores. Check it every time you go shopping to see if you need to make extra stops.

STEP TWO: Put things always in the same places. Do you spend time looking for things—glasses, tools, TV remote controls, pots and pans, foodstuffs, your automobile? This comes from habits formed when you were younger and automatically remembered where you had left your things. Now those patterns unnecessarily burden your memory when adopting several simple routines would eliminate the need.

1. Put a small basket or tray in each room for small loose objects. Always put glasses, TV remote controls, keys, and so on in that receptacle. You'll usually know exactly where to look for anything you've misplaced. If you have to hunt, a quick look in each room's receptacle will shorten the search.

2. Always park in the same aisle at the grocery store or mall. Maybe you'll walk a little farther than you would if you circled around seeking the closest spot, but you'll never suffer the embarrassment of having to hunt all over for your car. And if that aisle is full, the experience will be so unusual that you'll remember it.

3. Label shelves for foodstuffs and put up hangers for pans and knives. An organized kitchen unburdens memory both by making things easier to find and by making low supplies of staples obvious to help you assemble your shopping lists.

4. Hang tools on pegboard if possible. Then you never have to remember where you put them or paw through drawers and boxes hunting for them.

STEP THREE: Organize your finances. You can avoid the memory gaps that most often cause you real trouble by establishing routines for handling money.

1. Put all unpaid bills together. Keep each month's paid bills together, using large envelopes or rubber bands if you don't have a compartmented file. Check the previous month's bills before paying each new month's to avoid duplicating payments when bills and checks cross in the mails. Pay bills on the same day of each month to avoid either inadvertently failing to pay an important bill or paying bills twice. (These errors are the ones through which memory loss most often causes loss of independence.)

2. Ask for and keep receipts for any substantial cash payment. Keep these receipts in separate envelopes for each month.

3. Keep receipts from every credit card or open account transaction. Keep these in a separate envelope for each month, and review them if you think you have been charged for something you didn't buy.

4. Pay by check whenever possible, and keep all canceled checks.

5. Don't be ashamed to get help from a knowledgeable relative or friend. If you have followed these suggestions, anyone whose judgment you trust can get a clear picture of your finances quite quickly and easily.

STEP FOUR: Keep a detailed calendar. Write down everything you expect to do—social engagements, doctor appointments, meetings, and so on—on the same calendar, and check the next day or two's entries every morning when you get up. You'll avoid missed dates and conflicting engagements and also have a record to review. You'll find lots of use for old calendar pages, too. They'll help you to remember social obligations, names and places, and so on.

If you entertain in your own home, jot down details on your calendar. Later you'll be able to check on what you served the last time the Jones family visited, whether the Smiths have seen your new apartment, and so on.

STEP FIVE: Rolodex® like mad. Use a different card file system if you prefer; I don't own stock in Rolodex®. The main point is to record names, addresses, and phone numbers on convenient cards and to keep them very handy. Cards work better than address books because you can add any number, can sort them into categories (business versus personal, doctors, bridge players, or whatever), and can make changes or deletions. If you use categories, I suggest cross indexing or making duplicates; it's easier to jot down a name and number on an extra card than it is to remember whether you listed someone as a friend or a bridge player.

Mary S.'s son Jim wanted my advice on whether to get her admitted to a nursing home. He knew that she loved her independence, but wondered whether she could still handle living alone at age eighty-three. A recent incident worried Jim: He dropped in on his mother and found that she had run out of bread and meat. When he asked what she planned to eat she just answered vaguely, and he felt sure she just wasn't going to bother.

Jim and I went over the suggestions for taking the strain off memory that we've just discussed. He was willing to help with shopping once a week and to check back to see whether the previous week's purchases had been consumed. After two months he reported that the reorganized household had worked out well. His mother seemed to be eating regularly and had gained three pounds. Her finances were in better order, and she hadn't missed a single appointment or engagement. He felt completely comfortable about letting her continue in her own household.

PRIME STRETCHER 3

Improve your memory with multiple input channels.

Every teacher knows that visual aids, lecture notes, and recitations help students to learn. Each kind of signal your brain can receive, not only from senses like eyes and ears but from the motions involved in writing and speech, contributes to memory. Your brain records something you have *seen* and something you have *heard* or *written* in different ways. Each input channel adds to your chance of retrieving the fact or experience later.

Teachers deal mainly with long-term memory—the function that lets you store facts for much later retrieval. But the same principles affect the type of memory generally involved in stretching your prime: short-term memory. Aging doesn't usually have much effect on either long-term memory or instant recall (what you use when you look up a telephone number, then turn to the instrument and dial). The kind of memory it affects lets you recall the name of the person you met 5 minutes ago or street directions you have to follow after you've called and asked for them on the telephone.

STEP ONE: Repeat out loud everything you want to remember. Don't be afraid that people will think you're talking to yourself. In most social situations, it seems perfectly natural. Suppose, for instance, that a friend introduces you to a new acquaintance.

"Meet Harry Glitzman," he says.

Is there anything improper about saying: "Harry Glitzman? Glad to meet you!" instead of just "Glad to meet you"?

Checking back out loud does no harm. Most people are proud of their names, for instance, and appreciate your taking extra notice of them. Meanwhile, saying the name helps you in three ways:

- It makes sure you have your facts straight. What a shame if you struggle to implant "Glitzman" when the man's name is "Guzman"!

- Repetition helps memory. You're both *hearing* the name again and *speaking* it, which makes two more impacts to drive the message home.

- Speaking the name is a form of recitation. As an action, it uses different nerve pathways and reinforces input to memory.

Other apt moments for this technique are the following:

- Whenever you park your car. Just say something to yourself like: "Left side of second inbound lane to the right of Penney's entrance." When you get to the store entrance, look back and point to the car, repeating the same words. Follow this routine consistently and you'll never rove around and around another parking lot (unless you come out the store's other entrance).

- Whenever you get doctor's orders or other instructions that you want to carry out faultlessly. It never hurts to say, "Let me see if I've got this straight. I should _____ ." Saying it yourself not only checks the accuracy of your understanding but also helps your memory more than having the other person repeat the message.

- Whenever you get spatial directions. Remember the story about the farmer who sent a tourist on a long and complex route that led right back to his farm? "Wanted to be sure you could follow directions before I bothered" was his next remark. Probably the voice of experience, because a special kind of memory is involved in "right at the third light, left at the second, left again after two blocks." Such directions always end: "You can't miss it," which makes you feel all the more stupid when you do! Just repeat them out loud two or three times and you're less likely to have this experience.

- Whenever you make a date or appointment that you have to remember until you get home to your calendar. Just nodding your head when the other person says: "See you next Tuesday at 2!" doesn't engrave the date. Saying "Tuesday at 2? Got it!" helps.

STEP TWO: Write down crucial facts, or trace them with your finger on your thigh. Carry a pocket diary and pencil or pen and jot down anything you want to remember. If that isn't convenient, you can help yourself to remember by writing the key facts on your thigh with your finger. This gives memory input from the writing motions and from vision as you watch the movement.

If the circumstances don't permit these motions, you can get part of the memorization boost by closing your eyes and visualizing the name or entry while you move your finger (under the table, behind your back, or in your pocket) as if you were writing it. You can write "Glitzman" with your finger as if the paper were moving underneath it, for instance. The movements will hardly be noticeable and will really make it much easier for you to retain the name.

PRIME STRETCHER 4

Try to establish patterns and associations.

When I learned about the solar system, my teacher put this phrase on the blackboard: "My very educated mother just served us nine pumpkins." Sounds crazy, but I still remember the planets and their positions relative to the sun (Mercury, Venus, Earth, Mars, Jupiter, Saturn, Uranus, Neptune, and Pluto).

Just in case we might later get the two "M's" mixed up, my teacher went on to say that Mercury was what was in thermometers, all heat comes from the sun, so Mercury is the closer. You can use similar mnemonics or associations to aid your memory.

STEP ONE: Use established patterns and codes if they're available. If some of your activities involve short-term memory, see whether others have worked out suitable patterns or mnemonics like the following:

- A good contract bridge player keeps track of each suit by eliminating patterns of distribution. (If he sees five spades in his hand and three in the dummy, the other five are divided 0–5, 1–4, or 2–3. If everyone follows suit once, only 1–4 or 2–3 remain possible, etc.). He doesn't need to remember every individual card.

• Good gin rummy players often keep track of runs by constantly updating a four-digit code, one digit for each suit, each digit the sum of a 1 (for a low number), a 3 (for a middle number), and a 5 (for a high number). Instead of trying to remember every card that has been played, he might think "4199" (meaning that he's seen a low and a mid club [1 + 3], only a low diamond and a low, mid and high heart and spade).

• A knitter making a complex patterned sweater might use a similar code, perhaps consisting of the last digit of each number of similar stitches in a row, assuming common sense will take care of the ten column and that the second half of the row mirrors most of the first. She need remember only "4632" instead of "Knit 24, purl 16, knit 33, purl 22, knit 33 (backward from the central panel's 2), purl 16, knit 24"—quite a difference!

If no such established method exists for your own favorite activities, perhaps you can devise one. Devising and memorizing a code or mnemonic pattern uses long-term memory, which usually endures into your nineties, to unburden short-term memory, which often fades much sooner. Doesn't that make sense?

STEP TWO: Impress items into your memory with associations.
One memory training expert used to stand at the entrance of the lecture hall and ask everyone who entered his or her name. Later in his program, he would name anyone in the whole hall who held up his or her hand.

Although I suspect that this man had special capacities in addition to the technique to which he attributed his success, that technique certainly has merit. It involves visualizing some object that reminds you of the name and linking that image in your mind with a key element in the person's appearance.

For example, with the name "Rhodes" you can just visualize the man with a road cut through his hair.

Sometimes it's a bit more complex. Perhaps "Schneider" means "tailor" to you (that's what it means in either German or Yiddish), "tailor" suggests scissors and Mr. S. is totally bald. Your mind goes through all those steps in an instant and you imagine a barber snipping scissors futilely adjacent to Mr. Schneider's head. You'll remember his name for life!

Sometimes you might need to break a name into syllables and try to devise an image that links them together. For "Pascal" you might visualize a bear (Cal) throwing a football (pass) and seek a physical resemblance between the person and the bear. "Lowry" might turn into "Low Rye" with your image replacing his shoes with brown loaves of bread. "Rumpelstiltskin" would be no threat with this system, especially if he were tall and sloppily dressed.

Sometimes you need to work a "sounds like" or a pun into the process. Miss "Jones" might turn to "bones," especially if she's either very thin or very fat. "Descesceur" might turn into "The saucer," the memory consolidated by visualizing the woman balancing a saucer on her head.

Besides the associations themselves, this system makes you really think about each person's name. Especially if you have brief contact with a lot of people (in a sales situation, for instance), you'll find it very helpful. One caution: you'll have to develop a poker face if you use this system. Otherwise, the picture of baldies getting haircuts or husky women growing hair and throwing a football will cause facial changes that will make your new acquaintances think you are laughing at them.

CHAPTER
17

How to Free Yourself from Headaches

You can safely use home measures for some types of headaches common in the mature years and feel younger and more vigorous by ridding yourself of their misery.

A great many different conditions can cause headaches. In this section, I'll tell you what to do about several of the most common ones and how to recognize some varieties for which prompt medical care might be crucial. But I can't possibly cover all varieties. If you have other accompanying complaints like fever, burning on urination, dizziness, or nausea, or if the headaches persist or recur in spite of home measures, you should certainly see your doctor.

PRIME STRETCHER 1

Relieve cervical nerve root pressure pain with posture change or neck stretching.

One form of headache becomes more and more common after age forty: dull, steady (not throbbing) pain in the back of your head, never extending forward of your ears. Sometimes this is accompanied by brief twinges of sharp pain when you turn your head or look up and down or by burning or aching pain in one shoulder and upper arm. This kind of pain almost always comes from irritation of a nerve root.

The nerves that lead to the skin and muscles of the back of your head come from the top two segments of your spinal cord. As you grow older, wear and tear on spinal joints cause spurs to form that often press on the roots of these nerves. You can usually distinguish this kind of pain from any other by rubbing the side of a pin's point across your skin from the normal toward the painful area. The pin will suddenly feel distinctly sharper at the margin of the affected zone.

If cervical nerve pressure is causing your headache or shoulder-arm pain, these measures usually give relief:

STEP ONE: Try posture correction exercises. The spurs from arthritis press much harder on your cervical nerve roots when your neck bends back. Even mild osteoporosis (see Chapter 3) causes some bowing of the upper back, which forces you to increase the curve in your neck's spine to balance your head and look straight ahead. Slumped posture, often related to decreased muscle tone, has exactly the same effect.

Each curve in your spine influences the others. An increased hollow in your low back forces increased bowing of your upper back to keep your weight balanced, and increased bowing of your upper back forces backward arching of your neck. To straighten your neck curve, you need to take some of the curvature out of your entire spine. (*Caution:* Don't do this exercise if you have had a ruptured lumbar disc or low back pain that shoots down one of your legs. In these situations, you need to maintain the hollow in your low back to avoid any pinching between two vertebrae of the damaged disc, which is located at the front of your spine.)

1. With your heels about 8 inches from a smooth wall, lean back against that surface.

2. Put your hand into the gap between the wall and your lower back to see how much space is there.

3. Now try to reduce that space by two maneuvers:

- Lift the top of the back of your head as far as possible toward the ceiling.
- At the same time, tilt your hips forward.

4. When you have narrowed the gap between your lower back and the wall as much as possible, rock forward away from the wall and try to keep your head and back in the same position.

5. Repeat this many times a day until the straight spine posture becomes ingrained. This might be every 5 or 10 minutes the first day, less and less often as time goes on.

You will probably need about a month to establish the new posture thoroughly—longer if weak muscles need to be strengthened before you can improve posture to the maximum.

STEP TWO: Stretch neck muscles with head traction. Posture correction alone may not give full relief. Years of contraction let muscles set. Osteoporosis of any degree, even quite mild, causes inflexible bowing of the spine. Large spurs may still cause pressure even when you have perfect posture.

Nerve root pressure starts a vicious circle. The pressure causes pain, the pain causes spasm, the spasm causes more pain. You can break this circle by stretching the vertebrae apart for a few minutes at a time.

To do this, you need a device that pulls your head steadily to stretch your neck. You can buy "cervical traction equipment" from large drugstores or from dealers listed in your Yellow Pages under the heading Hospital Equipment and Supplies. This set should include

- A head sling

- A spreader (rod with hooks at its ends for the head sling's loops and an eyelet in the center for attachment to rope)

- Rope

- Pulleys on a frame that either hooks over the top of a door[1] or fits at the foot of your bed

- A sturdy plastic water bag

Buy a foot-of-the-bed rig if you have a spare room where you can ordinarily leave it set up. It's slightly easier to relax your muscles to allow the stretch to occur while reclining. The doortop unit also works reasonably well, though.

Assemble the set by attaching the head sling to the spreader and the spreader to the rope that runs through pulleys to the suspended water bag. Adjust the bed unit so that the pull tips your head slightly forward as it stretches your neck. If using a doortop unit, sit on a straight chair facing the door. Move the chair back until the pull tips your head slightly forward. *The muscles you want to stretch are at the back of your neck.* The device won't help you if it pulls your chin more than the back of your head.

Markings on the water bag show its approximate weight when filled to various levels. Your head weighs about 8 pounds, so you need at least that much weight to stretch your neck muscles. Start with that amount, stretching for 10 to 20 minutes once a day, to get used to the pressure. You can read, listen to music, knit, and so on during the treatment if you wish. Increase the weight as your tolerance builds. Don't expect much relief until you get to 12 pounds or more. Your outfit will probably handle up to twenty pounds, which should be more than enough to give relief.

When head, neck, and shoulder-arm pain have vanished, ward off recurrence by stretching once or twice a week.

---

[1] Perhaps I should say *sturdy* door. One of my patients visited his serviceman son in Thailand and stayed in a highly rated hotel. He hung his neck stretcher on the room's door. The door promptly fell in and remained unrepaired for the rest of his stay.

PRIME STRETCHER 2

*Relieve menopausal and vascular headaches
with caffeine and ibuprofen.*

STEP ONE: Control or prevent menopausal headaches.
Menopause-related hot flashes come from suddenly dilated blood vessels in your skin. A similar change in blood vessels inside your skull can cause throbbing or bursting headaches. A cup of strong coffee often gives instant relief. If that fails, one or two ibuprofen tablets (available at your drugstore without a prescription) should be effective.

If such headaches occur frequently, consider asking your doctor for menopause-fighting hormone pills or injections. As explained in Chapter 5, the positive effects of hormones more than balance their harmful side effects. This makes it sensible to use them for relief whenever you get substantial menopause-related complaints.

STEP TWO: Make migraine headaches less frequent.
Before age forty throbbing headaches accompanied by nausea generally turn out to be migraine. After age forty, migraines should become milder and less frequent. If they don't, you can usually help make them disappear by toughing out one or two without using any product containing ergot (such as Cafergot® tablets or ergotamine tartrate injections). Recent studies show that these products (which migraine sufferers have used for decades as the best nonnarcotic means of getting relief) have rebound effects that make the headaches recur much more often and continue for extra years. Stick to these mild measures for one or two attacks:

- Several cups of strong coffee
- Rest in a dark room
- An ice bag at the back of the neck
- 400 to 600 milligrams (mg.) of ibuprofen (two or three nonprescription-strength tablets). Prescription-strength tablets trade-named Motrin® may be stronger, so check the label.

Keep track of the frequency of migraines while following this program. You'll find that they become progressively less frequent and usually disappear by age fifty if ergot is avoided.

If you have never previously had migraines and develop headaches accompanied by nausea or vomiting after age forty, see your doctor right away. While that combination of symptoms can be from various mild disorders, it indicates serious disease often enough to deserve full study.

STEP THREE: Deal with vascular headaches. If you don't have nausea, mild throbbing headaches often yield to home measures. Since they occasionally show high blood pressure (especially if they occur first thing in the morning), you should check your blood pressure before using home measures. You can do this in either of two ways:

- By using the machine you'll find in many drugstores, either free or coin operated, for digital readout.

- By buying a home blood pressure measuring device. This is worthwhile if you or other members of your household have family members who have had high blood pressure or stroke. See Chapter 2 for detailed directions.

Your systolic pressure should be 140 mm. Hg or less, your diastolic 90 millimeters of mercury or less. Initial readings could be higher because of the emotional upset involved, but if your pressure settles into that range, your headaches certainly don't come from hypertension and you can safely try home measures.

1. Drink one or two cups of strong coffee.

2. Take two nonprescription-strength ibuprofen tablets.

3. Put a cold cloth or padded ice bag on the back of your neck for 10 minutes.

4. If you're not substantially well in half an hour, see your doctor.

PRIME STRETCHER 3

Relieve food- and diet-related headaches.

STEP ONE: Check for hypoglycemia. One of the easiest types of headache to identify and cure comes from low blood sugar, called hypoglycemia. Decreased food need, live-alone dietary neglect, and more frequent disorders of sugar metabolism make this condition more and more frequent as the years go by. These headaches don't throb: they build up steadily to "bursting" quality. You usually suffer from them late in the morning (especially if you've skipped or had a light breakfast), late in the afternoon, or as a reaction to sugar-controlling medications (usually taken for diabetes). The way to tell if such headaches are from low blood sugar is very simple: drink a glass of orange juice or eat a few soft Swedish mints. If your headache is hypoglycemic, relief is almost instantaneous: one of my patients clocked it as 40 seconds from misery to total comfort.

If you get hypoglycemic headaches, use sugar-containing foods like orange juice only to establish the cause of the pain or for emergency relief. Large amounts of quickly absorbed sugar kick your blood sugar up abruptly, setting in motion your body's sugar-storing mechanisms. Your body then usually keeps storing sugars until your blood sugar gets well below normal again. The immediate relief of headache is followed by recurrence in an hour or two unless you follow up with other foods.

Both as follow-up to relief from sugar intake and as prevention of future hypoglycemia, *foods high in protein* work best. Your body uses only a small portion of the protein you consume as protein, to repair or build tissue. You convert the rest to sugar with processes that take several hours. That's why protein foods like meat and cheese "stick to your ribs"—they produce a slow dribble of available sugar within your system for many hours, warding off hunger and also preventing hypoglycemia.

After relieving a hypoglycemic headache with orange juice or mints, eat at least one serving of a protein food (see box) within an hour to avoid rebound. I've emphasized foods appropriate for breakfast, because you can use this same list for preventing further hypoglycemia, and breakfast is the meal most likely to lack proteins. Egg whites (or an egg if your arteries can stand it—see Chapter 1) can be cooked with cubes of the meats mentioned to increase protein content. For prevention of future headaches, be sure to eat three meals a day and to include at least one serving of a protein food in each. In this respect, advertising often proves deceptive: three breakfast cereals advertised as "complete" averaged less protein per serving than one bite of turkey ham. Usually the milk you pour over your cereal has much more protein than the cereal itself—plenty to meet basic nutritional needs, but scarcely qualifying as protein foods for this purpose.

Convenient Protein Foods

Smoked fish (e.g., kippers)
Turkey ham or turkey pastrami
Chipped beef
Tuna (water packed)
Cottage cheese
Whole or partly skimmed milk cheeses (Edam, Gouda)
Eggs or egg whites

STEP TWO: Check for food allergy. Headaches from food allergy can be either throbbing or steady. Usually they involve the whole head. An unusual type of diarrhea often accompanies head pain—watery movements, beginning and ending abruptly, often with virtually no griping abdominal discomfort or malaise.

Although most other allergies (like hay fever and eczema) tend to get better in full maturity, food allergies become more common and severe as the years go by. If you suspect this cause of headaches, see if you get relief from nonprescription antihistamine preparations like Chlor-trimeton® 4-mg. tablets or Benadryl® 25 mg. If you can't obtain a pure antihistamine, use a tablet like Allerest® that combines an antihistamine with nose lining shrinkers. You don't need these extra ingredients, but unless you have high blood pressure, they won't hurt you.

If antihistamines relieve your headaches, see if you can figure out which food might be causing them. This isn't as easy as it sounds: the substance that spurs your symptoms usually forms in your system some time during the process of digestion. Often hours will pass between the time you eat and the time this substance forms. Occasionally, the offending substance forms only when you have eaten a large amount of the allergenic food. This happens when your body has different ways of digesting that food, some of which it only uses when preferable pathways are saturated.

For these reasons, you may need to collect considerable data before you identify your food allergies. Whenever you get an allergic headache (or diarrhea), write down everything you have had to eat for 24 hours. After several incidents, you may be able to pin down the cause of your trouble.

Most Common Food Allergens

Wheat, flour, cereals
Milk and dairy products
Eggs
Shellfish
Beans, including
    Kidney beans
    Peanuts
    Chocolate (cocoa beans)
    Soy beans
    Coffee

Notes: 1. True milk allergy differs from milk intolerance due to lactase deficiency. You can get allergic symptoms from cheese, yoghurt, and so on that would not affect you with milk intolerance.
2. Most people with bean allergy have symptoms only when the total intake of all different forms of bean passes a certain threshold.

If you can identify and eliminate (or keep below your tolerance level) the offending foods, your headaches will disappear. (See also Chapter 22.)

STEP THREE: Check for xanthine withdrawal. If you generally drink coffee, tea, or cocoa (or eat chocolate) every day, your system may have developed a true need for the stimulants these contain. You may get either a throbbing or a steady all-over headache from xanthine withdrawal. Coffee contains caffeine, tea both caffeine and theophylline, and cocoa theobromine. These are all xanthines, withdrawal of which can produce symptoms.

The test for withdrawal is very simple: see if consuming your usual amount of the missing substance cures the headache. Relief usually occurs within 5 minutes. Prevention is very simple: either keep up your xanthine habit or taper gradually.

PRIME STRETCHER 4

Relieve or prevent tension headaches with warm cloths, nonprescription medications, and progressive muscular relaxation.

Steady (not throbbing) aching all-over head pain generally comes from nervous tension. Discomfort tends to build up over a period of time rather than begin abruptly.

STEP ONE: Ease the pain with heat, massage and ibuprofen, aspirin or Tylenol®. Although you would swear that this pain originates deep in your tissues, it really comes from tight muscles in the scalp. Several measures generally give prompt relief:

- *Hot moist towels* applied to the whole scalp area for 10 minutes or so often help.

- *Gentle stroking massage* frequently gives relief. Stroke with limp fingertips from the top of the head downward with one hand moving toward your face and the other toward the back of your neck.

• *Ibuprofen, aspirin or Tylenol®* helps break the pain-spasm-more-pain cycle.

STEP TWO: Learn to use relaxation techniques. If you get this type of headache often, take time to learn progressive muscular relaxation and the refresher slouch (Chapter 15, Prime Stretcher 2). You can use these techniques to keep tension from building up until headache occurs.

PRIME STRETCHER 5

Ease sinus headaches.

If allergies and polyps have blocked off your sinuses in the past, you may continue to have trouble after forty (although these problems usually decrease with advancing age). Sinus pain starting in your mature years usually comes from completely different causes.

Most sinus pain hits just above the inner ends of your eyebrows. Sometimes a different sinus, located beneath your cheek bones, also becomes painful. Pain usually is steady but occasionally will throb. If pain in either location is accompanied by fever, enough infection is involved to make a prompt visit to your doctor worthwhile. Otherwise, home measures are worth a try.

STEP ONE: Improve sinus drainage with decongestants. Your sinuses normally contain air. They have openings into your nasal cavity that keep either pressure or vacuum from developing within the sinus cavities. Whenever those openings become plugged, sinus pain soon develops. If the cause of the stoppage is infection or allergy, fluid pours into the closed-off space, causing painful pressure. If the cause of the stoppage doesn't involve formation of fluid, your blood vessels carry away oxygen from inside the sealed-off cavity, creating a painful vacuum.

Unplugging your sinus openings relieves both these situations. Swollen blood vessels in adjacent nasal membranes have almost always caused the obstruction, so shrinking those blood vessels usually provides relief. You can accomplish this in either of two ways:

- Take decongestant tablets. These work by shrinking arteries all over your system, which means that they temporarily raise your blood pressure. If you have hypertension, do not use these pills. Otherwise, Sudafed® or Sinaid® will usually give considerable help.

- Use nose drops. This approach keeps most of the action confined to the vessels you want to shrink, so it has much less effect on your blood pressure. It works very well for *occasional* sinus discomfort. If used regularly for more than three days, though, rebound congestion almost always becomes a problem. After prolonged use, the drops shrink your nose lining for a few hours, then actually cause it to swell again. If you use more drops for the rebound congestion, you get into a vicious circle that can last for years.

For *infrequent* sinus pains, I recommend Neosynephrine® 1/4 percent nose drops (available without a prescription). Lie on your back with your head dangling over the side of the bed. Turn your head as far as you can to one side. Put two drops of Neosynephrine® in the *lower* nostril. Let it soak in for a minute or so; then turn the other way and put drops in the other nostril. Wait 5 minutes, then repeat *once only*. Go through this entire routine every 4 hours as necessary. (If you are unusually sensitive to this medicine, you may note fast pulse or light-headedness afterward. If these effects are very mild, cut back to one drop each time. Substantial side effects mean you can't use this medicine, of course.)

STEP TWO: Apply light bulb heat. Warmth soothes sinuses. Most people find light bulb heat easiest to apply. Just cover your eyes with moist cotton balls and shine the light from a 100-watt light bulb in a plain reflector on your face from a distance of about 1 foot. Adjust the heat by moving closer or farther away.

STEP THREE: Use Tylenol® for extra relief. One tablet or capsule of this commonly available nonprescription remedy every four hours helps to relieve sinus discomfort. Aspirin is also effective, but if you take aspirin for its artery-conserving effect you should avoid using it for other disorders (see Chapter 1).

STEP FOUR: Avoid future attacks with nasal moisturization. After age forty, your nasal lining becomes steadily thinner and drier. These changes interfere with the way your system normally deals with irritants and particles in the air you breathe. These unwanted materials normally catch in a microscopic layer of mucus at the surface of your nose lining. Tiny hairlike projections from the nose lining cells sweep this sheet of mucus back into your throat, where you swallow it.

As you grow older, the mucous glands and cilia become less active. Your nose lining (and the lining of your sinuses) becomes thin and dry. Irritants that you breathe in remain wherever they happened to settle. Some get into the sinuses themselves, where their irritation causes discomfort. Ultimately, trapped irritants cause sufficient swelling to close off the openings between the sinuses and the nasal cavity. The mild sinus headaches caused by irritation of the sinus lining turn into severe ones caused by pressure of trapped fluid.

You can nip these problems in the bud by keeping your nasal membranes moist.

Add humidity to heated air if possible. Every five degrees of added warmth lets air hold twice as much moisture. That cuts its relative humidity in half or (looking at it another way) doubles its drying power. Relative humidity of 70 percent or more keeps nasal membranes perfectly moist, but that is almost impossible to maintain in any heated space. Do what you can with pans on the radiators, humidifying devices in your furnace or cold fogging devices from your drugstore.

Use saline nasal spray. The products available at your drugstore do a good job, but the sprayers are made nonrefillable. That's all right if you don't mind paying for the convenience of ready mix. Two dollars or more for 1.5 ounces of a solution you can make yourself for a few cents a pint seems a bit stiff

Saline Nasal Spray

1 tablespoon glycerin
1½ tablespoonfuls rubbing alcohol
1 teaspoonful table salt
1 pint (preferably) distilled water

All ingredients are available without a prescription.
If you use tap water rather than distilled, let it stand in an open vessel for 24 hours to let chlorine escape.

to me, though. If you don't mind mixing your own, get a refillable atomizer at your drugstore or at a hospital supply store. Mix the solution as shown in the box.

A squirt of saline nasal spray in each nostril several times a day will keep your nose lining moist and help your nasal membrane to dispose of irritants. You'll find that it not only prevents most sinus discomfort but also eliminates nasal crusts and dryness-caused nosebleeds.

Nose lining ointment also helps to keep your nasal lining healthy and makes sinus headaches less likely. Follow this procedure about three times a week during the heating season and weekly in warm weather:

After using saline nasal spray to minimize crusts and other blockages to its spread, apply a gob of lanolin (no prescription needed) to each side of the wall between your nostrils about 1/4-inch up from the opening. As the lanolin melts, the microscopic hairlike protrusions from nose lining cells will spread it back to cover your entire nose lining. If lanolin is not available or if you find the smell objectionable, use *unmedicated* white petroleum jelly[2]. *Caution: Children under age twelve should never use any oily substance inside their noses.* This method is suitable only for adults.

---

[2] Vaseline® is the most common brand of petroleum jelly. The unmedicated form is fine, but the medicated type contains carbolic acid, which can harm your nose lining's tissue. This is less effective than lanolin, so you should use it about twice as often.

CHAPTER
18

Relieve Arthritis and Rheumatism the Natural Way

When you try to decide what makes someone seem old, the main physical change you think of is creaky, deformed joints. The passing years almost always bring some arthritis from wear and tear. This differs greatly from the red swollen joints caused in earlier years by rheumatoid arthritis. Joints may swell somewhat, but usually without redness and without fever. Finger joints may become knobby, but don't twist off toward the sides of your hands in the typical rheumatoid deformity.

"Wear-and-tear arthritis" generally smolders along without making joints red and swollen and without causing fever, loss of appetite, or other signs of general bodily illness. It usually makes you very stiff and sore in the morning, wears off as the day goes on, and then causes increasing misery as you become fatigued. You can control these problems and minimize later deformity with simple home techniques.

PRIME STRETCHER 1

Take the misery out of joints afflicted with smoldering wear-and-tear arthritis with paraffin baths, contrast baths, massage, weight shifting, and ibuprofen.

Paraffin baths give tremendous help for smoldering arthritis. They relieve pain and minimize later deformity. If you have enough joint trouble to spend an hour getting relief, try this method.

STEP ONE: Use paraffin baths for arthritic fingers. The joints of your body most likely to be affected by arthritis are those of your fingers. Almost everyone over forty has at least some knobbiness or lost flexibility there. If you have substantial pain or misery in these joints, paraffin baths give great relief.

1. Take off your rings. If you have heavy hair on the back of your hands, shave the area before your first treatment.

2. Heat 2 pounds of paraffin (from the canning supply section of your food store) with 1 pint of mineral oil (from your drugstore) in a double boiler.

3. When the paraffin has melted, remove it from heat and let it cool until a scum forms on top.

4. Dip your less painful hand quickly in the pool of melted paraffin. Dip again and again until the paraffin "glove" is about 1/4-inch thick.

5. Cover with a dry towel.

6. Dip your more painful hand as in step 4. When the "glove" is 1/4-inch thick, immerse the whole hand in the paraffin and leave it there.

7. Enjoy the soothing warmth for about 20 minutes.

8. Perspiration underneath the paraffin will have separated it from the skin. Peel it off and put it back in the pan. You can use the same mixture many times.

9. After several treatments, you may want to apply slightly more intense heat. If so, change the proportion of paraffin to mineral oil. The less mineral oil you put in the mixture, the warmer it will be at the time of application. Try 2 pounds of paraffin with 1/2 pint of mineral oil. After trying this several times, if you want an even warmer application use straight paraffin with no mineral oil at all.

10. Always let the mixture cool until a definite scum forms. Don't try to make it hotter by short-changing the cooling phase, or you might get burned.

11. Use this technique as often as necessary to gain relief. That will usually be once or twice a week, but more frequent paraffin baths won't hurt you.

STEP TWO: Use paraffin baths for arthritis of the shoulders, knees, hips, or back. You can also use paraffin baths for larger parts of your body by painting the paraffin on instead of dipping in it. Once again, we're talking about smoldering wear-and-tear arthritis, not abruptly inflamed red swollen joints. We'll talk about those later. If your shoulders, knees, hips, or back have become gradually more uncomfortable over a period of weeks or months, paraffin baths almost always help.

1. Shave the area.
2. Prepare, heat, and cool the paraffin as in steps 2 and 3 in the preceding list.
3. With a paintbrush with rubber or other hydrocarbon-resistant bristle setting material, paint several coats of the hot paraffin on the sore knees or the sore part of your back. Continue until the paraffin is about 1/4-inch thick.
4. Cover with a dry towel.
5. Enjoy the soothing warmth for about 20 minutes.
6. Perspiration underneath the paraffin will have separated it from the skin. Peel it off and put it back in the pan. You can use the same mixture many times.
7. Use the technique described in Step One to adjust the temperature as you become sufficiently accustomed to the heat to tolerate warmer applications.
8. Since much of the discomfort from large-joint arthritis comes from the vicious circle of pain-muscle spasm-more pain, paraffin baths once or twice a week (which break up that circle) usually give great 'relief.

If for some reason (like living in a room without adequate facilities) you can't take paraffin baths, a heating pad or hot compress gives some comfort. You should never lie on top of a heating pad and should use only the low setting to avoid any risk of burning yourself (especially if the pad becomes folded so that two wires cross).

If you have a number of sore joints, you might wonder why you can't just take hot baths or hot showers to get relief. Hot applications help joint troubles by increasing local circulation. If your whole body is hot, no part of it gets much of a circulatory boost. You can effectively treat two body parts at once, like both hands, both knees, an elbow and a shoulder, or a knee and an ankle. If you try to treat more than that at one sitting, you'll lose considerable effectiveness.

STEP THREE: Use contrast baths for joint or rheumatic pains of the hands, wrists, elbows, ankles, and feet. Next to paraffin baths, contrast baths offer the most effective home technique for soothing sore joints. Since contrast baths involve no special equipment, they generally prove more practical than paraffin baths for occasional miseries involving joints, muscles, bursas, tendons, and so on.

The pain nerves in all these structures run immediately adjacent to tiny arteries. Making those arteries alternately expand and contract is like putting massage right where the action is. Just follow this technique:

1. Assemble the needed equipment:

    * Two basins, plastic tubs, or wastebaskets large enough to accommodate the part to be treated
    * A thermos of very hot water
    * A bowl of ice cubes
    * If available, a candy or other accurate immersable thermometer
    * A book, magazine, or TV set to stave off boredom

2. Partially fill one basin with water at 105°F —moderately hot (not as hot as you can stand it) if you don't have a thermometer. Partially fill the other basin with 50° F water—as cold as it will run out of the tap in climates

harsh enough to require deeply buried pipes.[1] You should have enough water in each basin to cover the entire treated part, leaving room for the water your arm or leg will displace.

3. Soak the ailing part in the hot water for 4 minutes, then in the cold water for 1 minute. Continue to alternate on this rhythm for 1/2 hour. Always begin and end on hot.

4. Add hot water or ice cubes as necessary to maintain the temperatures.

STEP FOUR: Ease arthritis of ankles, knees, wrists, or elbows with massage. Arthritic pain comes from inflammation-caused congestion of the soft tissues supporting the joint rather than from the joint surfaces themselves, which have virtually no pain nerves. You can relieve that congestion by moving body fluids toward the heart with massage.

Massage works best if done by someone else, because it is easier to transport fluid through relaxed tissues and easier to relax if someone else is doing the work. Here's the technique:

1. Lie down and elevate the sore part on two pillows, arranged so that the lower part of the limb is level with the floor.

2. Apply mineral oil (or camphor and soap liniment if you prefer) to the area as a lubricant.

3. Get your helper to rub gently with his or her palms and limp fingers, stroking from the affected joint toward your heart, then lifting the hands off and stroking again in the same direction. Stroking should initially be very gentle, but should become progressively deeper so that it moves fluids out of the area's tissues. Stroking should continue for 10 minutes.

---

[1] When I moved to Florida from Minnesota, as I mentioned earlier, I used to let the water run and run, trying to get it cold enough to drink. I finally figured out that with no danger of freezing, the pipes aren't buried deep enough for the water to *ever* get cold.

4. Clean off the lubricant with rubbing alcohol and towels.

STEP FIVE: Spread or rebalance weight. When you have arthritis in any weight-bearing joint, including your spine, even a slight overload pushes the natural lubricant out from between the joint surfaces. The effect is like overloading a truck until the fenders scrape the tires: lots of extra wear and tear.

You can have this kind of problem without being even 1 pound overweight. If your legs aren't perfectly straight, for instance, your lower leg acts as a huge lever to crush surfaces on one side or the other of your knees together. The effect on the affected side of your knee joints can be the same as if you weighed an extra 100 pounds! Any difference in leg length tips your pelvis to one side. That makes your spine curve, which puts an extra burden on one side of your spinal column. A 3/4-inch leg length difference shifts the division of the burden between certain right and left joints from 50-50 to 60-40. The effect on the overloaded joints is the same as if you gained 10 percent of your present weight: 15 pounds if you weigh the average 150!

Changing your body alignment to balance your weight more evenly on available joint surfaces can thus *relieve* joint discomfort and *prevent* further wear-and-tear arthritis. Even if you have no knee or back pain now, alignment tests you can do at home might point to simple preventive measures that will save you years of misery.

To test your knees,

1. Stand erect.

2. Hold a piece of limp chain or a weighted string against the center of your kneecap and adjusting its length so that it just touches the top of your foot.

3. Mark the point at which it touches.

4. Measure from that point to each side of your foot.

5. Repeat for the other knee, which may not be the same.

If the measurement to the outer side of either foot is *less* than that to the inner side, your weight is crunching the inner side of that knee joint. You can distribute it more evenly by putting a heel wedge on the outer side of that heel. If the measurement to the outer side of either foot is *more* than that to the inner side, your weight is crunching the outer side of that knee joint. You can distribute it more evenly by putting a heel wedge on the inner side of that heel. You will need to wear Oxford-style laced shoes that fit your heel snugly or use heel counters to make the fit snug. Orthopedic shoes are ideal, but a good shoemaker can modify any low-heeled laced shoe at modest cost if you want to see what wedges do for you before making a major investment. If the measurement to the outer side of your foot is 1 to 2 inches different from that to the inner side, get a 1/2-inch wedge. If the difference is over 2 inches, get a 3/4-inch wedge. You won't be comfortable with ordinary shoes wedged up any higher than that. If the plumb line misses your foot altogether, it is quite likely that an operation to straighten your leg will prevent later crippling arthritis. You should consult an orthopedic surgeon.

To test leg length and its effect on your spine,

1. Tape a carpenter's level or a yardstick that you have established as perfectly level (by measurement, comparison with water level of a wide vessel or the like) to a wall mirror approximately at the height of the bottom of your chest. Have on hand two decks of playing cards or a stack of magazines.

2. Strip and press both thumbs into your sides at your waist line and slide them down until they hit the top of the pelvic girdle. Mark the site of the bony rims at these spots with a grease pencil, lipstick, or felt-tipped pen.

3. Stand with your back toward the wall mirror. Hold a hand mirror in your right hand and tilt it so that you can see your back. Move closer or farther away and shift the height of the hand mirror until the mark you made on your right side lines up with the top of the level or yardstick. Unless the mark on your left side lines up perfectly with the top of the level or

yardstick, put cards or magazines under one heel (usually the left) until your hips are perfectly level.

4. Measure the thickness of paper or cardboard required to level up the top of your pelvis.

There's better than a one in five chance that you'll find over 1/2-inch difference in leg length with this test. If you do, get a shoemaker to raise the heel of the appropriate shoe. The extra piece he puts in should be as thick as your shortness measurement at the back, tapering 1/8 inch at the front of the heel (so that the front edge won't catch on irregularities as you walk).

Bert T. complained of backaches that came on after he had been at work for an hour or two and got steadily worse through the rest of the day. At age fifty-five, Bert stood almost all day at his toolmaker's bench working drills and lathes, but he had enough seniority that he didn't ever have to lift anything heavy. Still, the discomfort was enough that he took Advil® or Tylenol® almost every day. He was seriously considering early retirement at considerable financial loss.

When I looked at Bert's back, I could see that he tilted a bit to the left. Measurement showed that his left leg was 3/4 inch shorter than the right. I suggested that he have a shoemaker put a lift on his left heel, which he promptly did. Two weeks later, he checked back telling me that his backaches had almost entirely disappeared.

STEP SIX: Lose weight if necessary. Even if your weight lines up perfectly on your various joint surfaces, you can get a lot of relief from pain in weight-bearing joints by shedding a few pounds. Having battled a bulging waistline all my life, I know how difficult this is. But many of my patients who had never previously been able to keep weight off have done so when they found that they got relief from painful joints.

STEP SEVEN: Take ibuprofen in six-day courses. Of the medications available without a prescription, ibuprofen generally gives the most relief from wear-and-tear arthritis. Ibuprofen works mainly by soothing inflammation rather than blocking pain sensation. To take full advantage of this action, you need to keep a steady level of the medicine in your bloodstream for several days. Moreover, this action accomplishes more if you use peak doses right away, before your tissues become accustomed to the product, than if you creep up on the dose. The creeping adjustment of dose lets tissues develop tolerance, so that when you reach larger doses, they aren't as effective as they would have been right away. I know that you want to use as little medication as possible to get relief, but in this case the way to minimize drug use is to hit hard at the start.

- If you weigh 150 pounds or more, take three 200-mg. (nonprescription-strength) ibuprofen tablets three times a day, after breakfast and lunch and with milk at bedtime. Taking ibuprofen with food makes its main side effects (nausea and heartburn) less likely.

- If you weigh less than 150 pounds, take two 200-mg. ibuprofen tablets on the same schedule.

- Unless you get side effects (which are unlikely with this schedule) continue full doses for six days even if you feel completely well.

- After six days, cut down by one tablet at each dose for three days. If symptoms recur, resume the higher dose. If relief persists, lower your daily dose by one tablet every two days (cutting the noon dose first, the morning dose next). Continue to use paraffin baths and massage simultaneously, in the hope that they will help you get away from medications altogether. If joint pains again become troublesome, take full doses of ibuprofen for two days, and then drop to the smallest dose that previously gave adequate relief.

PRIME STRETCHER 2

Keep alert for signs of gout.

The most common cause of red, swollen joints after age forty isn't arthritis: it's *gout!* Big toe pain isn't really characteristic of gout as the Katzenjammer comic strip might have made you think: only one patient in every ten has this complaint. Any joints can be involved, including large ones like knees and elbows. And gout isn't punishment for overindulgence in high living: it hits as many teetotalers and beer drinkers as gourmands.

Because of all these misunderstandings (and because the blood test on which many doctors depend doesn't become constantly positive until many years after onset), you have an excellent chance of futilely treating yourself (or being futilely treated) for arthritis when you actually have gout.

STEP ONE: Keep a detailed food and symptom diary. If you get gout, your body ceases to dispose properly of breakdown products made from purines. Purines are proteins contained in many foods (see the accompanying box).[2] In the course of utilizing purines, your system makes uric acid. If excessive amounts of uric acid pile up, they form sharply pointed crystals. Movement makes these tiny crystals scrape and puncture surrounding tissues.

Since at first formation of the crystals rids your bloodstream of the excess uric acid, measurement of that substance in your bloodstream gives normal readings by the time you have joint pain. Your doctor can't prove that you have gout unless you happen to have a test just before an attack is due. (Here in Florida we have a fish that strips bait off the hook so fast that natives say you need to set the hook just before the first nibble. Testing for gout works that way, too.) You may suffer

---

[2] Perhaps this is the source of the idea that gout is associated with high living. In poorer cultures or older times, only the rich could afford enough protein foods to get gout. That is not so today.

High-Purine-Content Foods

Organ meats
Brains, kidney, liver, sweetbreads
Seafood
Anchovies, herring, mackerel, mussels, roe, sardines, scallops
Meat juice products
Bouillon, broth, consommé, gravy, soups
Miscellaneous
Mincemeat, partridge, yeast

Moderately High-Purine-Content Foods

Meat, fish, shellfish, and poultry not included above
Asparagus, dried beans, lentils, mushrooms, dried peas, spinach

---

for as much as ten years before the blood test remains constantly positive.

You can often do better with common sense and a food diary than your doctor can with his or her laboratory. Just keeping track of what you eat and studying your food diary for the week before two or three attacks may make you highly suspect gout.

STEP TWO: Confirm the presence of gout if possible.
Checking to see if aspirin gives more relief than ibuprofen or Tylenol® (see recommended dosages shortly) gives another clue. I don't like to use aspirin for relief of joint pain because this interferes with the artery-sparing method I hope you adopted after reading Chapter 1. However, aspirin does have distinct uric acid-removing qualities besides its anti-inflammatory and pain-relieving actions. This makes it work better than ibuprofen or Tylenol®—so much so that the difference stands out as a diagnostic test. Don't take aspirin if you have had peptic ulcers

or internal bleeding. Otherwise, take one pill for each 50-pound body weight after each meal and (with milk) at bedtime for two days. If you get dizziness or nausea cut back to half doses. If the attack subsides promptly, taper one pill per dose every two days.

Deliberately precipitating an attack with a day or two of very high-purine intake is a painful but often effective way of telling whether you have gout. If an attack occurs but there's still doubt in your mind, try again after a couple of weeks and get your doctor to take daily blood tests for a week while you're eating a high-purine diet. Usually the level of uric acid will go up and then subside just before you get joint pains.

STEP THREE: Try a low-purine diet with aspirin. Home treatment of gout involves a very stringent low-purine diet. You should eat no more than 2 ounces of meat a day, avoid gravies and soups altogether (stocks derived from protein foods have high concentrations of purine), eat no vegetable that is the seed of its plant (like beans and peas), and avoid all organ meats like liver and sweetbreads.

One aspirin after each meal and at bedtime helps to make the diet more effective in warding off joint symptoms. This dose aims at moving uric acid out of your system, not effectively fighting inflammation. If you get an attack, you'll need the larger doses detailed earlier.

STEP FOUR: Get your doctor involved. It is worthwhile to involve your doctor whenever you think that you might have gout. Safe prescription medicines quickly move uric acid out of your system. This lets you eat a much more liberal diet without precipitating symptoms. A rigid low-purine diet works very well, but it really disrupts your life-style—you almost have to prepare your own meals separately, which disrupts both your family life and your social life. Prescription medicines won't relieve your need to avoid purines altogether, but they let you eat enough of them to live a reasonably normal life.

PRIME STRETCHER 3

*Relieve muscular rheumatism and stiffness
with special massage and hot showers.*

Every time a muscle contracts, it makes lactic acid, which is a distinctly irritating substance. When a muscle contracts very often or very intensely, it makes a lot of lactic acid. Ordinarily, lactic acid moves out of your tissue by way of lymph passages. Juices always flow slowly in these tiny, thin-walled vessels, but movement becomes even more sluggish as your circulation slows with the passing years. It takes longer and longer to carry away all the lactic acid formed by any muscular exertion. This irritant piles up in your tissues, causing stiffness and aching pain. (For applications to foot and back miseries, see Chapters 11 and 18.)

STEP ONE: Move acids out of aching muscles with fingertip massage. You can speed lymph flow, move waste products out of the over-wrought muscle, and rid yourself of stiffness and muscle pain in several ways. Here is one effective technique:

1. Press the tips of your fingers very firmly into the painful muscle.

2. While maintaining pressure, move your finger in circles as far as the elasticity of your skin readily permits for about 5 seconds.

3. Release the pressure. Move your finger to an adjacent portion of the sore muscle and move as recommended.

4. Continue until the pain goes away, showing that you have kneaded the acids out of all sore areas.

Concentrating pressure on the small surfaces of your fingertips helps transport accumulated acids into and through lymph vessels. Those vessels work like sponges: squeeze the liquid out, and they'll soak up more irritating acid instantly! But it takes considerable pressure to empty them, and some muscles (like those of your back) are hard to reach. That's where this next technique comes in.

STEP TWO: Use heavy-impact shower massage. Shower massage combines improved circulation and muscle relaxation through heat with multiple lymph vessel-compressing impacts. It works very well on back pain. You need to adjust the shower massage device for heavy, pounding action.

Follow this technique:

1. Remove any flow restriction devices from your shower, and install a head with capacity to deliver firm pulsations.

2. Adjust the temperature toward the hot side (heat helps to relax the muscles, so that their tension doesn't block transporting action of pulse impact).

3. Drape a towel over your back so that the shower comes through it. (That holds the heat and makes it more effective.)

4. Stand with both knees bent and both hands resting on your knees, with the pulsating shower striking through the towel to the sore muscles.

5. Move your hips as if you were drawing figure eights with your rectum, so that the muscles alternately contract and relax.

6. Continue for about 10 minutes (if the hot water holds out).

PRIME STRETCHER 4

Soothe inflamed tendon sheaths with splinting, ibuprofen, and contrast baths.

Once you're past age forty, repetitive movements tend to make the tendon sheaths in your wrists become inflamed. You paint your bathroom walls or work in the garden with a trowel and the next day your wrist and forearm really hurt. If you hold the sore area against your ear and move your fingers, you hear the tendons creak as they scrape against inflammation-roughened sheaths.

Inflammation does roughen those normally supersmooth surfaces, making every motion cause friction, which causes still more inflammation. You can break up this vicious circle in two ways: by avoiding motion and by combatting inflammation.

STEP ONE: Splint or rest both the sore wrist and the corresponding fingers. The tendons in your wrist move literally inches when you flex and extend your fingers. If you get substantial pain in your wrist and forearm, you need to restrict motion of both the wrist and the fingers to keep those tendons from grating against inflamed sheaths. The best way to do this is with a splint.

To keep your fingers still, grasp a roll of gauze bandage or two men's handkerchiefs rolled into a cylinder. Lay a thin wood slat or a medium-thickness magazine along the top of your wrist. Get a helper to apply a 3-inch elastic bandage to keep these objects in place. Keeping the bandage always under moderate stretch, your helper should wind two anchor turns around your wrist, bandage all sides of your fist, then spiral up your forearm to secure the upper end of the splint. Leave this in place for three days, while taking ibuprofen (discussed shortly). If movement still hurts when you take the splint off, reapply it for three more days. If movement remains painful after following this program for six days, see your doctor.

If for some reason splinting is totally impractical, try to rest the hand and wrist as much as possible. Keeping your arm in a sling helps to remind you not to use it unless absolutely necessary. If you must use it, try to keep your wrist stiff and to grasp objects between straight fingers or between a straight thumb and the side of your hand. These motions don't use wrist tendons.

STEP TWO: Take ibuprofen. Take one 200-mg. (nonprescription-strength) ibuprofen tablet three times a day. You'll be using this for its anti-inflammatory action, not to relieve pain. That means that you should take it regularly whether your wrist hurts or not until two days after you remove the splint and stop having pain on motion.

Actually, the main drawback of using ibuprofen is its pain-relieving quality! When you don't have pain to warn you, it's easy to use the ailing part before it has completely healed. Don't let the ibuprofen-induced freedom from pain lure you into resuming activity too soon, or you'll have to start from scratch again.

STEP THREE: Use contrast baths. Contrast baths (see Prime Stretcher 1, step 3) work very well for tendon sheath inflammation. If your helper doesn't mind reapplying your splint over and over or if you aren't using a splint, try to work this technique into your schedule once a day. It will definitely speed healing.

PRIME STRETCHER 5

Combat bursitis with pressure bandaging,
ibuprofen, and heat.

When two adjacent structures have to glide smoothly along one another in your body, a bursa often forms. Besides the one already mentioned in regard to bunions (Chapter 11, Prime Stretcher 3), bursas that commonly cause pain are located near your kneecaps, elbows and shoulders. These bursas are smooth-walled collapsed sacs like empty balloons. Normally, they contain only a few drops of lubricating fluid, but when inflamed (in bursitis), they fill with blood or fluid. This ordinarily happens after either repeated movements or repeated pinching against a hard surface (e.g., when you do a job like scrubbing the kitchen floor on your knees).

If substantial swelling occurs before you get started with home measures, you will get well much more quickly if you see a doctor right away. Once the bursa is filled with blood or fluid, getting those irritants out with a sterile needle helps a lot. But if you can use them immediately, home measures can control the condition.

STEP ONE: Put on a pressure bandage right away to minimize accumulation of fluid in the bursa.   At the first sign of discomfort at the front of the knees or near the point of the elbow, put on a pad of gauze bandage or a folded handkerchief and a snug elastic bandage. If practical, lie down and elevate the part on two pillows. These steps will keep down the amount of fluid that forms inside the bursa and speed healing.

STEP TWO: Take ibuprofen in full doses for three days. Once again, you'll be using ibuprofen for its anti-inflammatory action, not simply for pain relief. To make this effective, you should keep a level of the medicine in your bloodstream at all times. That means taking two tablets (or three if you weigh over 180 pounds) three times a day. Continue for at least three days even if the pain disappears promptly. You still need to keep the inflammation soothed for at least two days after tenderness disappears to prevent reaccumulation of the fluid.

STEP THREE: After swelling begins to subside, use heat. Heat increases circulation through a part. Don't use heat in the early phases of bursitis: increased circulation at that point just makes more fluid fill the bursa. Once your body starts to reabsorb instead of pour out fluid, however, heat helps your system carry it away. If the area can easily be immersed (like an elbow), soak it in hot water (112°F if you have a candy or other immersable thermometer) 20 minutes three times a day. Otherwise, use hot wet towels, changing them as often as necessary.

CHAPTER
19

How to Reverse Age-Related Back and Neck Conditions

The part of your body's framework that shows the most change with age is your spinal column. The muscles that support it become weaker and impregnated with fibrous strands that limit their capacity to stretch. Every vertebra in your neck and back has four joints, the edges of which develop spurs as you grow older—spurs placed where they often push on adjacent nerve roots. The intervertebral discs, which are cartilage pads between the bodies of your vertebrae, squash down and become less elastic. The vertebrae themselves may weaken and collapse from osteoporosis (see Chapter 3). You can limit or reverse many of these age-related changes with the methods and techniques in this section.

PRIME STRETCHER 1

Transport lactic acid out of aching back muscles.

As mentioned in the last chapter, every contraction of a muscle fiber forms lactic acid. Lymph vessels soak this up and carry it away, but age-slowed circulation often fails to keep up. If lactic acid accumulates in your tissues, you get aching pain. Also, in the long run, acid irritation makes strands of fibrous tissue form in muscle, shrinking it and making it less elastic.

269

STEP ONE: Prove to yourself what lactic acid removing massage can do by using fingertip massage for driver's neck-base pain. The best demonstration of the lactic acid effect I know occurs when you take a long drive, especially on bumpy roads. Every bump and jolt jostles your head, and muscles at the base of your neck have to contract to keep it balanced. After an hour or so, these muscles begin to ache like a toothache.

Fingertip massage as described in Chapter 18 gives instant relief. You won't believe how fast the pain vanishes until you try it! And please do: that will convince you of how much good you can do for yourself with the other forms of acid-removing massage I'm going to suggest.

(Before we leave the subject of driver's neck-base pain, let's take a look at prevention. If you readjust the whiplash-preventing headrest on your seat and your body position so that your head presses firmly against the headrest, the jiggling motions that strain your neck-base muscles on long rides will be damped out. You'll find that long rides are much more comfortable.)

STEP TWO: Have a helper roll away overworked muscle pain. You can literally "roll away the pain" of a work-weary, aching back. Virtually all muscular backaches come from lactic acid accumulation, which you can eliminate by squeezing out the fluid from the spongelike lymph vessels. In heavy back muscles, that takes more pressure than you can manage with your fingertips. If you have a willing helper, use this technique:

1. You'll need a 2-foot length of 1-inch x 10-inch smoothly finished wood, adhesive tape, and a tennis ball.

2. Wrap two or three thicknesses of tape around the board near each of its ends. Your helper will be holding on and pushing down on those areas, so they need to be smooth and slightly cushioned.

3. Lie on your stomach on a firm surface. (The floor works better than a soft bed.)

4. Have your helper kneel astride your knees.

5. Get him or her to put the tennis ball underneath the center of the board and against the middle of your worst aching muscle.

6. Get your helper to lean against both ends of the board, putting pressure on the tissue beneath the tennis ball.

7. Get your helper to move the board so that it rolls the ball along and across the aching muscle, moving acids into the lymph vessel "sponge."

8. As the pain disappears from each area, ask your helper to move up, down, or across until all the ache-generating irritants have been transported out.

This technique works very well if your helper can exert (and you can tolerate) enough pressure to eliminate the accumulated acids. But particularly if you're overweight, the tennis ball may give sufficiently intense pressure to be uncomfortable. In that case, use a larger ball, such as a seamless softball. Your helper will have to lean a little harder to make the less concentrated pressure suffice. If this still causes discomfort, use a softer ball, like a children's rubber ball the same size as a softball.

STEP THREE: Roll pain away yourself if you don't have a helper. Here's a modification of the previous technique to use when you don't have a helper:

1. Pick a smooth, solid wall that can't be damaged by a tennis ball, even when you're leaning hard against it. If you don't have a suitable wall handy, buy a piece of Masonite® for reinforcement.

2. Stand with your feet about 12 inches apart and with your heels about 18 inches from the wall.

3. Put a tennis ball between the wall and the center of one of your sore back muscles.

4. Lean solidly against the ball.

5. Bend your knees and roll your shoulders to move the ball across and along the sore muscle, always maintaining heavy pressure. You will probably have to arch

your back to bring the involved muscles into contact with the ball.

6. When you have "rolled the misery" out of one side of your back, put the ball near the center of the aching area on the other side of your spine and repeat the process.

7. Try a larger or softer ball after you have experienced the relief that a tennis ball can give. By leaning harder (since the pressure is spread over a larger area), you may be able to get similar relief more quickly.

STEP FOUR: If the foregoing methods are impractical, try closed-fist massage. If you have a willing helper, use this method:

1. Lie on a firm surface, where your helper can comfortably reach (and press firmly on) your back.

2. Get your helper to spread some mineral oil over the area.

3. Get your helper to close both hands into fists and use the flat surfaces of the second finger segments to press firmly into your aching muscles near the base of your spine; then (maintaining the pressure) slide both fists up along your back muscles to the rib cage.

4. Get him or her to repeat this action 10 or 12 times, varying the site slightly to cover the entire width of the lengthwise back muscles.

5. Your helper should then open the fists and stroke with firm fingertips diagonally from the center of your lower back toward both sides of your rib cage.

6. Finally, he or she should wipe off the oil with rubbing alcohol, which leaves you feeling extra clean and refreshed.

If you don't have a willing helper and are strong enough to press hard on your own back in a clumsy position, you may be able to transport those backache-causing acids for yourself. Here's the technique:

1. Sit on a straight chair.

2. If practical, bare your back and lubricate with mineral oil. (This makes it easier, but you can still get some relief massaging through a layer of cloth.)

3. Ball both hands into fists. Lean forward and reach around with both arms to press the backs of your knuckles into your back muscles as high up as you can reach.

4. Continuing pressure, slide your knuckles down to the base of your spine.

5. Repeat several times, until your back ache disappears.

PRIME STRETCHER 2

Deal with stiff neck with heat, ibuprofen, and self-manipulation under traction.

Some serious disorders, including meningitis and stroke, involve stiff neck. If you have other symptoms like headache, fever, or dizziness with a stiff neck, you should call your doctor.

After age forty or so, you may find that sitting in a draft makes you get a stiff neck. This condition probably starts with spasm of the arteries rather than the muscles, but the pain starts the usual vicious circle of pain-muscle spasm-more pain.

STEP ONE: Treat sporadic stiff neck with heat and ibuprofen. If you can catch a stiff neck at its start, a hot towel will often relieve the blood vessel spasm before the muscle pain-spasm cycle begins and give instant relief. Once the stiffness is fully established, heat still helps, but further measures are usually required. A single nonprescription-strength (200 mg.) tablet of ibuprofen usually helps.

STEP TWO: For perpetual stiff neck, try self-manipulation under traction. Over a period of years, the muscle spasms involved in occasional stiff necks sometimes cause permanent changes. Firm strands of fibrous tissue within the muscles keep them from stretching, and the tightness actually sets off further muscle spasm.

If this happens, a perpetual stiff neck results. You need to stretch those muscles and restore their elasticity. Use this technique:

1. Obtain and set up a head traction device as described in Chapter 17. Start with 8 to 10 pounds of water in the bag, and be sure that the direction of pull is such that your head stays tipped forward and your chin stays down.

2. Stretch the muscles for 10 minutes before attempting the manipulation.

3. Turn your head far to the right. Place the heel of your right hand against the left side of your chin and gently press straight back.

4. Turn your head to the left and press back with your left hand.

5. Repeat steps 3 and 4 three times with gradually increasing (but never really hard) pressure.

6. Do this daily for one week. If stiffness hasn't abated, see your doctor. If it has, carry out this technique once a week to avoid recurrences.

PRIME STRETCHER 3

Ease shoulder-arm pain from pressure on nerves passing through your neck by easing compression.

If you squeeze on a tube of toothpaste, the paste squirts out at the end, not where you exert pressure. Pressure on a nerve shaft works similarly. It causes pain where the nerve ends rather than where the pressure actually occurs.

When that pressure strikes nerve roots leaving through the top two segments of your spinal column, you feel the pain in the back of your head, as discussed in Chapter 17's Prime Stretcher 1. Pressure on other nerves in your neck cause pain in your shoulder and arm, where those nerves end. Two different age-related conditions create such pressure. If you get such pain, you need to sort out the cause before picking appropriate home measures.

STEP ONE: Test yourself for a narrowed thoracic outlet. The nerves leading to your shoulder and arm pass through a very narrow passage between the heads of the scalene muscle and the first rib at the base of your neck. They share this narrow space with the main artery leading to your arm. Age-related changes in the artery often make it easier and easier for pressure to irritate the nerves.

A simple home test tells you whether you have (or might later have) this problem.

1. Locate the pulse in your wrist. Lay your left index and middle fingers across the front of your right wrist with their tips near the heel of your hand at the base of your thumb. You feel the pulse better with the pulp of your fingers than with their tips. Make sure you can feel it easily.

2. Raise your right arm straight out to the side of your body, then bend the elbow so that your forearm points straight forward.

3. Try to feel the pulse in your right wrist. If you have a narrow thoracic outlet, the pulse will either be very faint or totally absent.

4. Follow the same procedure with your left arm.

STEP TWO: Don't wait until you have pain to take steps if you have a narrow thoracic outlet. If the pulse test reveals narrowness of either thoracic outlet, take appropriate steps right away. Three measures help to avoid future shoulder-arm pain.

- Avoid any work above your head. Not only will your arms become numb from blood vessel pressure if you try to do a job like painting the ceiling or putting up acoustic tile, but the irritation that results from pressure on nerves may cause pain and misery that goes on for months.

- Avoid pillowing your head on your arm when you sleep. You may even need to break the habit of sleeping in this position by wearing a tether for a few weeks. Some of my patients have done this, wearing a belt around their chests with a felt cuff for the arm and a length of cord between the two. They leave some slack for comfort, but not enough to let them raise their arms more than a few inches.

- If you get shoulder-arm pain anyway, put hot wet towels where the pressure occurs, above your collarbone at the base of your neck, rather than where you feel the discomfort. Keep the towels hot for 20 minutes, and repeat three times a day until the pain disappears.

STEP THREE: Treat shoulder-arm pain with head traction if the thoracic outlet test shows no constriction. If you have no narrowing of the thoracic outlet, shoulder-arm pain almost always results from pressure on nerve roots as they emerge from the spinal column. The spurs formed by wear-and-tear arthritis through the years tend to impinge on these nerves. The proper corrective measures are exactly the same as those I described for a headache caused by similar nerve pressure at a slightly higher level in Chapter 17. The posture correction exercises and head traction techniques discussed in detail starting on page 238 work very well. Even after you get relief, you will need to continue the head traction once a week or so to avoid recurrences.

PRIME STRETCHER 4

*Control low back pain with weight loss or
rebalancing, ibuprofen, heat, massage, and
sleep support.*

No matter what makes your back hurt, several simple measures usually help.

STEP ONE: Change body balance or lose a few pounds to relieve back pain. Each of the dozens of joints in your spine has just a drop of lubricant in it. Extra weight pushes that lubricant out from between the joint surfaces and lets them grind together. Loading a joint until this happens is like loading a truck until the fenders scrape the wheels: the last little bit of weight causes a lot of extra damage. You can both relieve present discomfort and prevent considerable wear and tear by keeping this from happening.

Rebalancing your weight keeps certain joints or parts of joints from being overloaded. Check to see if your legs are slightly different in length with the technique described in Chapter 18 and use heel wedges (also described there) if necessary.

You may have found *losing a few pounds* very difficult in the past, but it's worth another try. Many of my patients who couldn't keep weight off have found that they could manage when extra weight and extra pain proved strongly linked.

STEP TWO: Take ibuprofen on an inflammation-fighting schedule. If you have constant or daily backaches, you'll get a lot more relief from ibuprofen if you use it to control inflammation instead of waiting until you have pain. That's like putting on an asbestos suit instead of putting out the fire. Ibuprofen controls inflammation much better with *high initial doses tapered promptly* than with doses that start small and build up as you need more for relief. To use this approach, it's also important to *keep a certain level of medication always in your system*. You can't get good effect by omitting medication until you have pain.

The right dose schedule for this purpose is the same as described for wear-and-tear arthritis, in Chapter 17.

STEP THREE: Ease back pain with paraffin baths or light bulb heat. The most effective home remedy I know for back pain is a paraffin bath. You'll find complete directions in Chapter 18's Prime Stretcher 1, Step Two.

If this procedure is impractical because you lack a helper, light bulb heat gives some relief.

1. Sit backward on a straight chair with your back bared.

2. Arrange one (or preferably two) lamps 12 to 18 inches from your back, shining toward it. If your lamps do not have metal reflectors, either use bulbs with built-in "spot" or "flood" reflectors or line the shades with aluminum foil to reflect and concentrate the beams.

3. Let the warmth penetrate and soothe your back for 10 minutes or more. Move the lamps closer to or farther away to adjust the heat.

STEP FOUR: Get a helper to give gentle stroking massage. Proper massage often helps to relieve arthritic back pain. Gentle stroking moves lymph out of the passages into which fluid from congested joints must move. (The deep, lymph-mobilizing kneading you use for work-weary muscle aches won't help here. The spine's joints lie too deep, and they are located in hard, unyielding tissue.)

1. Lie on your stomach on a firm surface that your helper can easily reach without bending.

2. Get your helper to lubricate your back with mineral oil.

3. He or she should use the surfaces of all four fingers on each hand and both palms and should stroke gently and rhythmically from the base of your spine toward your head. Each stroke should be 10 to 12 inches long. It should begin and end with very light pressure, with mild but distinct pressure during the midstroke.

4. Every stroke should begin and end 1/2 to 1 inch or so farther toward your head. This will ultimately cover your entire low back.

5. This pattern should be repeated two or three times.

6. Then your helper should clean off the oil with rubbing alcohol.

STEP FIVE: Get relief with proper sleep support. If you sleep on your back on a firm surface, the weight of your midsection tends to flatten the curve in your low back throughout the night. This stretches tight muscles, interrupting the vicious circle of muscle spasm-pain-more spasm.

A Japanese sleeping pad (futon) on the bare floor or a rigid platform makes an almost ideal support. If you have a bed with a coil spring and cotton mattress, putting a piece of plywood between the spring and mattress helps. Cover the edges of the wood with adhesive or packaging tape to avoid getting splinters under your nails when you make the bed. An innerspring mattress is the last choice, but if that's what you wind up with, get it as firm as you can tolerate.

PRIME STRETCHER 5

Prevent future back pain with appropriate exercises, according to the types of trouble you have had in the past.

Once you have relieved all or most back pain with these measures, you can take exercises to keep your trouble from coming back. You can't really start on exercises as long as you have much pain, because the accompanying spasm makes the necessary movements almost impossible.

STEP ONE: Decide which set of exercises is right for you. Let's sort out low back troubles into *rear-of-spine* and *front-of-spine* problems. Spinal joints, muscles, and ligaments all are located near the rear of your spine. The vertebral bodies and intervertebral discs lie toward the front. With the first kind of problems, you should take exercises aimed at *straightening* your low back— flattening its concave curve shifts your weight from the back of the vertebrae toward the front. With the second kind, exercises aim at maintaining and supporting your spine in its concave curved position, so that no movements concentrate your weight on the front part of your vertebrae.

For practical purposes, the only conditions that call for maintaining the concave curve in your low back are *ruptured and bulging intervertebral discs*. If you have reason to believe you have one of these, like those listed here, you should take concave curve maintaining exercises as described in Step Four. Otherwise, any low back problem you might have will almost certainly improve if you take these low back spine-flattening exercises.

Signs of Disc Troubles

Pain going down leg

Severe spasms of pain

Abruptly sharper sensation when you drag the side of a pin point across skin from painless to painful area

Past CAT scan evidence of ruptured or bulging disc

Past disc surgery

Past X-ray evidence of ruptured or bulging disc

STEP TWO: If you have no sign of disc trouble, spine-flattening posture correction exercises can help keep you clear of future back troubles. The more your lower back curves, the harder its muscles have to work, the more weight falls on its facet joints, and the more prone it is to ligament strains. When your spine is almost straight, vertebrae sit on top of each other like a stack of blocks. It takes very little muscular effort to keep them there, and both work-weary or arthritic backaches and ligament injuries are much less likely. I already described the proper *posture correction exercises* in Chapter 17, but they are so important that I'm going to repeat every word here:

1. With your heels about 8 inches from a smooth wall, lean back against that surface.

2. Put your hand into the gap between the wall and your lower back to see how much space is there.

3. Now try to reduce that space by two maneuvers:

   • Lift the top of the back of your head as far as possible toward the ceiling.

   • At the same time, tilt your hips forward.

4. When you have narrowed the gap between your lower back and the wall as much as possible, rock forward away from the wall and try to keep your head and back in the same position.

5. Repeat this many times a day until the straight spine posture becomes ingrained. This might be every 5 or 10 minutes the first day, less and less often as time goes on.

You will probably need about a month to thoroughly establish the new posture—longer if weak muscles need to be strengthened before you can improve posture to the maximum (see the discussion that follows).

This method prevents or makes milder most muscular and arthritic backache and makes you less subject to injury. Actually, I used this very exercise myself for posture correction long before I had to worry about stretching my prime. I was a medical student at Johns Hopkins and backed against a wall when I learned about this technique. I found that I could put my whole fist in the gap behind my lumbar spine. I did exactly what I've suggested you should do: walked away from the wall 20 times a day at first, then less and less often. In six weeks, I could hardly get one finger into the gap, and my back has stayed straight without further effort ever since.

I'm sure this has saved me a lot of discomfort and quite possibly some injuries (because a straight back is more stable as well as stronger). It can do the same for you if you're willing to spend a few hours *now* to avoid possible weeks of pain later.

STEP THREE: Strengthen your abdominal muscles to flatten your low back curve further. You'll also find that building up the strength of your abdominal muscles helps to straighten and support your back. Although these are lighter than your back muscles, they have the rib cage above and the pelvis below as levers.

When polio raged, victims whose abdominal muscles were paralyzed sustained much more curvature of the spine than did those whose back muscles were hit. This shows just how much *back* support your *tummy* muscles give.

Plain old flab can make your back hurt two ways: by contributing to extra curvature and by leaving your spine without muscular support. These abdominal exercises really help:

1. Skip this step if your tummy muscles are in pretty good condition. If your abdominal muscles have become really loose, start by just lying on your back and raising your head ten times. Do this four times a day for three days. Then go on to the next step.

2. Lie on the floor with your knees bent to a 45˚ angle and your feet hooked under a heavy piece of furniture. Lock your hands behind your head.

3. Draw your body into a sitting position. Let your upper body slowly back down onto the floor. This is called a straight sit-up. Repeat five times.

4. From the same starting position, touch your right elbow to your left knee. Let your body back down to the floor. Touch your left elbow to your right knee. This is called a turning sit-up. Repeat five times.

5. On the next day, perform straight and turning sit-ups six times instead of five. Increase by one repetition a day until you reach thirty.

6. If at any time you find your abdominal muscles sore, remain at the same repetition level for three days.

7. Continue to do thirty repetitions of each exercise daily.

STEP FOUR: Take an entirely different set of exercises if you have had disc troubles or back pain running down your leg. It's equally important to strengthen your abdominal muscles whether or not you have had disc troubles, but when you have had such problems, replace Step Three's exercise with one that lets you strengthen those muscles without any possibly painful or injurious back movement.

1. Lie on your bed. Bend your knees and plant your feet flat on the bed surface. Place the heel of each hand on the corresponding knee.

2. Lift your head off the bed. Push your right hand hard against your right knee for 10 seconds. While still keeping your head raised, push your left hand against your left knee for 10 seconds.

3. Let your head fall back and rest for 10 seconds.

4. Repeat five times.

You should do this at least twice a day, when you go to bed and when you wake up. One virtue of this exercise: you don't have to build up the number of repetitions. As you get stronger, the intensity of each contraction will increase, automatically suiting the effort to your capacity.

When you have a ruptured or bulging disc, you want to shift weight from the front part of your vertebrae (where the discs are) to the back—exactly the reverse of what I advised earlier for people who have never had disc troubles. The next set of exercises aim at establishing that posture. Stretching exercises play a big part in establishing new posture, and muscles stretch well only when they are warm. Therefore, you should always exercise your whole body by walking, riding a stationary bicycle, or the like before each session.

Before your pelvis can tilt forward to shift weight to the back part of your lumbar vertebrae, you need to stretch the muscles at the back of your thighs and those of your calves. That's the aim of this first set of exercises:

1. Fold a towel until it is eight or ten layers thick.

2. Lie on the floor with your left hip close to a door jamb, with the folded towel underneath your lower back.

3. Stretch your left leg up along the door jamb.

4. Press your knee to straighten your leg totally.

5. Relax and repeat three times.

6. Shift to the other side of the door and repeat the procedure with your right leg.

7. Next, stand facing the wall at arm's length.

8. Put both hands on the wall.

9. Move your left foot back about 2 feet.

10. Keeping your left knee straight, bend your right knee so that your weight presses your left foot up toward your shin, stretching your calf muscles.

11. Repeat three times.

12. Follow the same procedure with your right foot back.

You don't need to wait until you have fully stretched your thigh and calf muscles to start on the following exercises, that try to establish for you patterns of body movement that never pinch the disc area between two vertebrae:

1. Kneel on all fours.

2. Place a rolling pin lengthwise along your lower spine.

3. Without making the rolling pin move, simultaneously lift your right arm and your left leg level with your body.

4. Return to starting position. Simultaneously lift your left arm and right leg. Return to start, and repeat three times.

5. Next, learn to lift and stoop by bending your legs instead of your back using a broomstick or mop handle.

6. Hold one end at the back of your neck with your right hand.

7. Hold the other end against the base of your spine with your left hand.

8. Do a deep knee bend without letting your lower back get any closer to the stick than it is when you are upright. Repeat three times (and try to use exactly the same technique whenever you stoop or lift).

These exercises help a lot. You should do them twice daily and continue them until the patterns of movement have been thoroughly ingrained.

CHAPTER
20
How to Build Your Lung Power

How can you feel in your prime if you're huffing and puffing or stopping to catch your breath?

You can't, and that makes lung power a key to feeling and acting younger than you are. You can use respiratory exercises to restore or build your wind (and to stop smoking cigarettes, if you haven't already taken that step). If your loss of wind stems from aging or from residual damage of past disease or indulgence, simple exercises and home procedures that take only a few minutes each day often turn back the aging clock by many years. Ridding your home of airborne irritants also often helps breathing capacity.

Before using these home techniques, you should be sure that you don't have a currently active disorder (like a heart condition or bronchial infection) for which a doctor's prompt care is crucial. Breath-building measures might help you even if the weakness stems from high blood pressure, heart disease, or a bronchial condition, but you should use them to *supplement* rather than *replace* sound medical treatment. A thorough checkup in your doctor's office generally proves worthwhile whenever

- You lose your wind from unhurriedly climbing two flights of stairs or less.

- Shortness of breath comes on at night while you are lying flat, and forces you to sit up or go to the window for more air.

- Swelling of the ankles, bluish lips or dusky-hued fingernail beds, a feeling of pressure or constriction at the bottom of your breastbone or other signs of possible heart disease develop along with breathing difficulty.

- Cough (or change in the character of your cough if you have had a mild hack), pain in the chest, spitting of blood, or other signs of possibly serious lung disease develop along with lessened wind.

You need not be frightened if you have these complaints. They quite commonly come from innocent, mild, or readily cured conditions. But disorders that a doctor's care can greatly benefit cause these difficulties often enough to make prompt medical attention for them distinctly worthwhile.

PRIME STRETCHER 1

Improve your wind by helping the bellowslike action of your ribs and diaphragm.

Most age-related loss of wind comes from impairment of the bellowslike action through which you draw air into your lungs. You pull air into your lungs partly by pulling your ribs up into a higher, more flared position and partly by drawing downward the muscular sheet that separates your chest from your abdominal cavity. As the years go by, however, your ribs tend to remain in a higher, more flared position all the time. Their starting point on any one breath comes closer and closer to their peak, so that their movement draws less and less air into your lungs.

STEP ONE: Increase rib movement with this chest squeezing exercise. Here's an exercise that helps overcome the excess flaring of aging ribs and also helps empty pockets of mucus or pus in your lungs:

1. While sitting erect in a straight chair, place both hands flat on your lower chest and upper abdomen, with about one hand's breadth separating them.

2. Take in a breath normally; then let it out.

3. At the end of the air's normal escape from your lungs, press with both hands to expel abruptly as much air as possible.

4. About every third breath, press very vigorously and sharply, in the equivalent of an artificial cough.

5. Don't get discouraged if this exercise makes you cough. That means it is transporting mucus out of pockets in your lung and is giving extra benefit. Keep your hands as flat as if they were pressing on a table top—if you let your fingers dig in even a little bit, they will make your trunk muscles sore.

6. Continue for about ten breaths, and do this exercise three times a day.

This exercise gives special benefit if you have suffered the ravages of asthma, bronchitis, emphysema, or other lung disease, but also benefits the fixed, overexpanded chest brought on by the passage of time alone.

STEP TWO: Mobilize ribs further with the bend and breathe exercise. Here's another exercise that helps rebuild your breathing capacity by improving rib movement.

1. Stand with your back against a wall, with your heels 12 to 15 inches away from its base so that your hips press gently against the wall's surface. Let your arms hang loose.

2. Bend your head forward until your chin touches your chest, simultaneously letting your breath out gently and unforced. Gradually droop down so that your spine curls slowly away from the wall starting at the top and working down to your hips, allowing the compression of your chest and upper abdomen to squeeze

more and more air from your lungs as your body bends.

3. Let your arms and hands hang loose from your shoulders throughout the movement.

4. When you have bent as far as seems comfortable, gradually uncurl your body. Keep your abdominal muscles drawn in at first, both to make your breathing correct and to allow the lower part of your back to make first contact with the wall.

5. Let air flow into your chest without deliberately drawing it in while you straighten the rest of your body, bringing your low back, the back of your chest, your shoulders, and your head into contact with the wall. Do not tip your head backward to make it touch—keep the back of the top of your head high to maintain proper neck position.

6. Take a small breath without expanding your chest; then start the next bend.

7. Repeat six to ten times.

Besides making your ribs move less, age also tends to make the bottom of the bellows (your diaphragm) less efficient. When this muscular structure contracts, it moves from a high domed position up inside your chest to a flat disc at its bottom. The elastic recoil of your lungs then draws it back into its domed position. As the years go by, the flare of your ribs, weight of attached organs below, and loss of elastic recoil in your lungs make your diaphragm flatter and flatter. That leaves less and less range of possible motion. These exercises tend to restore its normal curve:

STEP THREE: Restore your diaphragm's curve and strength by breathing against sandbag pressure.

1. Fill a sturdy plastic bag with 10 pounds of sand (15 pounds if you weigh more than 150).

2. Settle yourself comfortably into a bed or on the davenport, lying on your back. Use two pillows under

your head if that aids comfort, but keep your backbone horizontal. Lay the sandbag on your lower abdomen, keeping it entirely below your belly button.

3. Place both hands against your lower chest and upper abdomen. Breathe in and out *without moving your chest wall any more than absolutely necessary*, using your diaphragm rather than the muscles of your chest. This will make your upper abdomen bulge out slightly whenever you draw air in.

4. Once you get the feel of it, you will find that you need not devote any particular attention to the process, and can read, knit, or watch TV to stave off boredom. Continue this form of breathing for 20 minutes on the first session and work up to a half hour or more over a period of two or three weeks.[1]

STEP FOUR: Mobilize and learn to breathe mainly with the better preserved core section of your lungs. When you were young, the chambers in your lungs had more surface area exposed to the air you breathed than a football field. That amount of surface area came from countless tiny air chambers. To understand how this works, think about a palace with many rooms. If you had to paint the *interior*, you would need many times more paint than if you painted the *exterior*. Every inside wall, partition, and ceiling adds area to the original bounds.

Both age and certain disorders make certain of these tiny chambers merge, losing forever the surfaces of their former partitions. This forms fewer, larger compartments from the numerous small ones, and thus decreases the surfaces through which oxygen can soak into your blood. If the loss of partitions becomes extreme, the condition becomes known as *emphysema*.

Both the merging of air chambers from the aging process and the more severe loss of emphysema (often precipitated by smoking, asthma, or chronic bronchitis) occur mainly near the

---

[1] If you're the 1 person in a 100 with a diaphragmatic hernia, this exercise can cause heartburn or indigestion. We'll discuss that condition in the next chapter.

outer edges of your lungs. The core areas near your diaphragm generally remain fully effective. The following exercises help to bring those portions of your lungs into play more actively when you breathe because *diaphragmatic breathing* draws air into the still healthy core areas of the lung.

First, loosen your lung's core section with recoil breathing.

1. Lie on your back in bed or on a comfortable davenport, with your knees slightly bent and your feet flat on the supporting surface.

2. Place both hands on your upper abdomen. Let your muscles go loose as if you were a rag doll.

3. Breathe out slowly but completely, letting first your chest and then your abdomen sink in. Let yourself go completely loose, so that air sucks into your chest by recoil action of your tissues without drawing it in deliberately.

4. Repeat ten times, then rest for 1 minute and repeat ten more times.

Second, increase ventilation of your lungs' core areas with the core-of-the-lung wind regainer. Here's an exercise that really comes into its own when you get short of breath and need to recover quickly—but you need to practice beforehand so that you'll be able to use it in time of need.

1. Either lie down or sit back in a comfortable chair that supports your back. Let your chest and abdomen relax completely.

2. Now draw in your abdomen rather sharply, forcing air out through your mouth or nose. Then let your abdomen relax again, reinflating your lungs. Each phase should take about 1 second, so that breathing this way continuously involves about thirty breaths a minute—half again the usual relaxed breathing rate.

3. Continue for 2 minutes (if short of breath, continue until your wind is restored).

Next, try pursed-lips or candle-blowing respiration. To get much use out of the core section of your lungs, you need to keep open the air passages through which they are ventilated. When you were younger, those passages were held open by the elastic recoil of the tiny partitions on all sides of them. With loss of those partitions (and loss of elasticity in lung tissue), only the air pressure inside those tiny tubes keeps them from collapsing when surrounding tissue presses against them. Since this inevitably occurs when you breathe out normally, no air escapes. On the next breath, the trapped air keeps fresh air from entering, and key parts of your lung become useless to you.

You can prevent this sequence of events with this technique:

1. Lie on your back. Breathe in *quietly* through your nose, using your diaphragm instead of your chest muscles. Your chest should remain virtually stationary, with the expansion occurring in your upper abdomen only.

2. Now pucker your lips as if you were blowing out a candle, and blow your air out through the reduced opening (letting the extra pressure puff out your cheeks).

3. After a few breaths in the reclining position, stand up and lean forward about 45°. Continue to breathe in quietly with your diaphragm and breathe out by blowing through well-puckered lips.

4. Gradually straighten your body, continuing the same mode of breathing. At first, you will find that you shift to rib-lifting rather than diaphragmatic respiration when your body is almost erect. Bend again until the proper pattern is established and straighten up once more.

5. Continue for about 10 minutes, getting your body as straight as possible without shifting back to the old way of breathing.

6. Do this every day until you have learned to breathe in quietly with your diaphragm even when standing erect and to breathe out by blowing at extra pressure through puckered lips.

7. Next time you begin to lose your wind, deliberately shift to this mode of respiration for quick relief. Or even better, breathe this way when performing feats that (in recent years anyway) often make you lose your wind.

Hilda G. had suffered lung damage from asthma when she was young. When osteoporosis led to chest deformity, breathing became so difficult for her that she needed to keep an oxygen tank with her wherever she went.

The word "exercise" scared Hilda off at first. She didn't see how she could tolerate the least bit of exertion. But when she read over the directions for the exercises I've just explained, she could see that they didn't call for much muscle effort and agreed to give them a try.

After six weeks, Hilda was able to leave her oxygen tank behind most of the time. She still carried it to the grocery store where walking and bending to pick up items from low shelves sometimes used more oxygen than her crippled lungs could deliver. But she felt completely comfortable without the oxygen at home, when she went to play bridge with friends, and on other relatively quiet visits. Just not having to carry the tank around with her doubled the amount of activity she could tolerate.

PRIME STRETCHER 2

Fight the cigarette habit with breathing exercises, especially if emphysema has made it harder for you to quit.

If you smoke cigarettes, the action of the smoke on your lungs changes your breathing rhythm. Immediately after a cigarette, you breathe more frequently and more deeply. You then tend to breathe gradually less often and more shallowly. You smoke another cigarette and start the cycle over again.

Your breathing never becomes so inefficient that you lack oxygen and feel short of breath. But your lungs not only provide your body with oxygen: they also rid your system of numerous gaseous waste products. The discomforts that make you "need a cigarette" are exactly the same as those that occur when a number of people gather in a poorly ventilated room and breathe in each other's noxious wastes.[2] While a few smokers (one study claims 17 percent) may be addicted to nicotine, many more simply need the extra blood purification that will come with smoke-spurred breathing. This seems especially true of people with emphysema. Even though this condition is often caused (and always made much worse) by smoking, people with emphysema have an even harder time getting away from the cigarette habit than anyone else. Reason: their damaged lungs have no reserve capacity for ridding their systems of noxious wastes.

A great many of my patients, including emphysema sufferers who had tried unsuccessfully a dozen times before, have been able to quit cigarettes with breathing exercises. These help smokers to get away from tobacco need due to inadequate clearing of noxious wastes until their breathing patterns readjust. Here's the technique:

1. Before trying to quit tobacco, do a simple breathing exercise at least three times a day. Put your left hand on your hip, your right on your tummy and stand erect. Breathe in through your nose, at first without raising your chest. Only after your lungs are as full of air as you can get them by moving the diaphragm, which pushes the tummy out under your hand, should the chest begin to rise. Fill your lungs further by expanding your chest, to their total capacity. Let the breath escape through your mouth.

2. Do this ten times.

---

[2] Other people's noxious wastes proved deadly in the Black Hole of Calcutta incident. Many people who read accounts of this incident thought the deaths were due to lack of oxygen, but an oil lamp continued to burn throughout. It takes 16 percent oxygen to support combustion, and people don't smother at that oxygen level.

3. Repeat the whole procedure at least three times a day.

4. After three weeks, quit smoking but *continue the exercises* several times a day, and also every time you get the urge to smoke, for at least three months.

5. Use any other helpful measures you have found, like gum chewing or eating extra crackers, along with the breathing method. And expect to gain some weight. Most smokers gain about 20 pounds when they quit, then lose about 10 of it within a year. (About half the gain is from replacing smoking's oral activity, which ends after your system adjusts. The rest occurs because nicotine impairs digestive efficiency, so when you quit using it, your system extracts about 10 percent more nourishment from every bite. That means that if you keep eating the same amount the nourishment provided will be the same as if you were eating 10 percent more and still smoking.)

Brad S. could hardly climb one flight of stairs without stopping to get his breath because of emphysema. Every doctor he had seen for years had warned him that cigarettes were making his condition worse. He had tried a dozen programs for quitting tobacco, including nicotine chewing gum, a therapy group, acupuncture, and hypnotism. None of them took, so he was very skeptical about the breathing exercise program. But the other methods in this chapter seemed sensible to him, and he figured while he was at it he might as well try the quit-smoking regime too.

You've probably guessed the outcome. The other exercises substantially extended his activity range, to the point where he could even play a round of golf (riding a cart, of course). And the quit-smoking exercises helped him kick a three-pack-a-day cigarette habit!

PRIME STRETCHER 3

Prevent later loss of breathing capacity by controlling cough and keeping mucus out of your lungs.

A good part of the loss of wind people blame on age actually comes from damage done by partial mucus plugs in the smallest bronchial tubes. These plugs often act like valves, letting air into the tiny chambers beyond when the bronchial tube is expanded during inspiration but trapping it when you breathe out. The trapped air builds up in pressure until it ruptures the super-thin walls of the tiny air chambers. You can substantially stretch your respiratory prime by keeping this from happening.

The three main causes of mucus plugs each call for different measures.

1. The answer to *smoke irritation* is obviously to quit smoking if you haven't already done so and to avoid smoke generated by others as much as is practical.

2. The answer to *infection-caused mucus* is to see your doctor promptly for any cough accompanied by fever over 100°F, to control cough with mucus-thinning rather than cough-inhibiting products, and to clear mucus out of your lungs with postural drainage and proper sleep position.

3. These measures also help *allergic attacks*, but you can also often add home measures to help control the underlying allergy.

STEP ONE: Quit smoking. If the future risk of early heart attacks and lung cancer hasn't convinced you to quit smoking, maybe something you can detect *right now* will be more effective. Get your doctor to run breathing tests on you. If you've been smoking for ten years or more, they're almost 100 percent sure to show the kind of damage we've been talking about through this whole chapter. The method in Prime Stretcher 2 will help.

**STEP TWO: Use mucus-thinning cough syrups and prep-
arations to help clear your lungs.** Cough syrups and loz-
enges labeled "expectorant" thin the mucus in your nose, throat,
and lungs. My own favorite preparation is Robitussin®, which
you can buy at any drugstore without a prescription. Stick to
plain Robitussin® rather than the products with added codeine
or other ingredients. Or if you prefer a generic, check the ingredients for names starting with "guai." Robitussin® has
guaifensin, others guaicolate or similar derivatives, all of which
have the desired action.

These products make a cough looser instead of keeping
it from happening. Codeine-containing cough products keep
you from feeling the "tickle" that starts the cough reflex. This
actually lets extra mucus accumulate in your lungs. While codeine
may help you to fight infection when used to help you get
enough sleep, unnecessary use may contribute to cumulative
lung damage. Expectorants actually help preserve your lung
power through the years, cough-inhibitors harm it, so use the
latter sparingly and preferably only at night.

STEP THREE: Rid your lungs of mucus with postural drainage.
Whenever you have any condition that causes cough, mucus
may be getting into your lungs. While the cough itself moves
out a great deal of the mucus, assuming a posture that lets
it run out under the force of gravity both decreases your need
to cough and rids your lungs more effectively of the mucus.

Perhaps the simplest form of postural drainage is *sleeping
on your stomach* when you have a cough. When you lie on
your back, your windpipe slopes 15° downhill *into* your lungs.
If you turn over, mucus runs out of your lungs instead of
down into them. This step alone usually keeps the small amounts
of mucus that you form with an ordinary cold or mild allergy
out of your lungs. You can make breathing easier if necessary
by propping one side of your body up a few degrees with a
pillow under one side of your chest.

Conditions that form larger amount of mucus or other
secretion such as bronchitis, bronchiectasis, and asthma usually
call for more intense drainage-promoting efforts. Whenever you

can hear or feel secretions rattling around in your chest, use this method of postural drainage:

1. Take a full dose of Robitussin® or other expectorant. Give this about half an hour to become fully effective.

2. Lie on your stomach across your bed. Scoot forward until only your hips and legs are on the bed. Let your upper body hang down at a 45° angle or more. Support yourself with your elbows on a footstool or hassock if necessary for comfort.

3. About every 30 seconds, take a deep breath. Cough whenever you get the urge. About every 5 minutes, shift your position slightly so that first one side then the other of your chest is slightly higher than the other.

4. If you have a willing helper, get him or her periodically to lay one hand flat on your rib cage just below your shoulder blades, then thump the back of that hand with the other fist. This will transmit a mucus plug-dislodging impulse without any risk of damaging your ribs.

5. Continue for about 15 minutes or longer if you are still raising considerable material.

6. Go through this entire routine shortly after arising every morning and before going to bed at night as long as your cough remains productive.

STEP FOUR: Eliminate common allergens and airborne irritants from your home. Whether or not you have had asthma or other allergic disorders in the past, dust, molds, and pollens aggravate mucus formation. When you have a chronic cough from any cause whatever, you can get some relief by eliminating as many of these airborne irritants as you can from your home, and particularly from your sleeping area.

"Removal" in this instance always means with water or oil. A dust cloth tends just to rearrange the dirt, and an ordinary vacuum cleaner bag lets a large share of the tiniest particles (unfortunately including most pollens and irritants) through.

Unless you have an expensive water-type vacuum cleaner, you'll need to follow these directions:

Get rid of all dust. You'll probably need to get a professional with a special machine to clean out the air ducts in your heating and air-conditioning system. Sponge away all dust (and associated pollens) from hidden corners of your living quarters. (If you have substantial allergies, get someone else to do this for you.) All drapes and curtains, hangings, and rugs should go into the wash, to the cleaners, or out in the yard for beating, home dry cleaning, or shampoo. All pictures, framed mirrors, and the like should be taken down, washed, and sponged off. Go over the furniture—top, bottom, outside, and inside—with an oiled or damp cloth. Remove and sponge every item from closets, cupboards, and bookshelves.

Once the original cleanup has been done, you can probably keep ahead of dust accumulation for a year or so if you follow my other suggestions for keeping new dust out of your house. If you use an ordinary vacuum cleaner, always get someone else to empty the bag (somewhere outside your house!). Never sweep or dust dry surfaces: if you want to sweep, soak torn bits of paper in water and scatter them liberally on the surface to be cleaned or use an oiled sweeping compound. Hit all dust-collecting surfaces in one room or area each week, taking different parts of the house in rotation, to supplement your ordinary weekly cleaning. If housecleaning makes your cough distinctly worse, perhaps you can trade chores with someone else in the family.

Dispose of dust catchers and holders. Stuffed toys, big rugs in the bedrooms, and lined drapes that need dry cleaning are dust traps. Replace them with washable toys, scatter rugs, and either lighter washable window dressings or fiberglass ones.

Settle irritants out of the air. Airborne dusts and pollens have very small particles, but they will ultimately settle out of *stationary* air. So decreasing air motion in your house helps free the air of irritants. That means windows closed tight and doors shut promptly both winter and summer. Oil-type furniture polish and oil-containing sweeping compound also help keep down dust by ensnaring it.

Filter out dust and allergens. An air conditioner or (even better) an electrostatic air filter removes almost all airborne irritants. If you get your doctor to recommend such equipment before you purchase it, you may get some tax advantage.

Seal dust-blowing cushions and springs. The biggest dust traps in your house are probably the cushions, enclosed springs, mattresses, and pillows. Every time you sit or lie on these, they act like bellows blowing puffs of irritant into the air. The very least you should do is cover or replace any unsuitable pillows and mattresses. Even if you aren't allergic to feathers, a soft pillow gives out puffs of dust and pollen every time you compress it. A foam rubber pillow and mattress eliminate this problem. Plastic pillow and mattress covers are almost as good. The thin plastic from dry cleaning, patched together with masking or packaging tape, makes a reasonable temporary way of seeing whether sealing yourself off from airborne irritants helps enough to make more costly arrangements worthwhile. For overstuffed furniture, a layer of oilcloth or plastic underneath slipcovers helps. A sheet of light linoleum tacked to the bottom of each piece of overstuffed furniture also helps.

Seal dust and pollen out of your living quarters. You can't clean all the dust out of attics, cellars, and storage spaces, but you can seal these spaces off from your living quarters. Especially if you have a damp basement (where molds often form and throw off airborne spores), a roll of masking tape to seal cracks around cellar doors will often make quite a difference.

Check chemicals. Many substances, from nail polish remover to floor wax, can irritate your lungs. Formaldehyde escaping from insulation or particle board causes a great deal of trouble in new or remodeled houses. If you find that your lungs clear up when you're away from home for a few days, check for this condition. Otherwise, try packing away all the dispensable chemicals in a sealed storeroom for a week to see if you feel any better.

Finally, consider giving away your pets and posies. A cat or dog can be a great companion, but if you are allergic to its dander it can also inadvertently cause untold later misery. Animal dander permeates the furniture and rugs sufficiently that you can't usually learn whether it is causing you problems just by sending the pet away for a few days. You can do a patch test (see the accompanying box) that will reveal a really bad allergy. Milder allergy may show up only on tests done by an allergist with injection techniques.

Animal Dander Patch Test

Part the animal's hair to get down to bare skin. Open a Bandaid® and hold the exposed pad adjacent to and below the bared skin. Holding a single-edged razor blade perpendicular to the skin, scrape several flakes onto the Bandaid® pad. Attach the Bandaid® to your skin between your shoulder blades and leave it in place for 48 hours (unless your skin becomes inflamed under it earlier). Check for inflammation daily for three days and occasionally for three weeks. If redness occurs, you need a different species pet.

You can usually tell whether house plants are aggravating your condition by taking them to a friend's house for a week or so.

CHAPTER
21
Quick Healing for Injuries

This story has happened so often that I can't attach one patient's initials to it:

(S)he led an active, enjoyable life until age fifty something. Then (s)he injured an ankle or other joint. By the time it healed, (s)he had been inactive too long to resume previous activities without an arduous retraining program, which (s)he kept putting off. By the time (s)he came to me, a sedentary life had led to restricted movement, lack of muscle tone, and resignation to "being past it," which combined to make it almost impossible for him (or her) to get back to the pre-injury activity level and physical capacity.

You can keep from falling into this trap. If an injury interrupts your activity pattern, you can take steps *right away* to keep it from dooming you to the rocking chair. Proper first aid can minimize the damage. Exercises help you to retain capacities during injury-enforced idleness. Prompt rehabilitation techniques get you back into action faster. And adaptive rehabilitation can often restore or find suitable replacements for lost capacities.

PRIME STRETCHER 1

Minimize damage with first aid.

When promoting one of my earlier books, I appeared on Garry Moore's TV program "To Tell the Truth," where several impostors pretended to be me. In preparing for the program, one of the impostors asked what he should say if asked how to treat any disorder.

"Put ice on it," I said.

When the program went on the air, the panel had virtually decided that one imposter was really "Dr. Eichenlaub" when Orson Bean asked him what to do about high blood pressure. The answer "take ice cold showers" (which several members of the panel knew would do more harm than good) promptly lost the game and forced the producer to make an emergency announcement cautioning viewers that treatment measures recommended by impostors shouldn't be used.

If Bean had just stuck to injuries instead of asking about disease, our team would almost certainly have won. *The right first aid for almost every injury is ICE!* Cold applications limit damage from sprains, strains, bruises, torn muscles, and even (along with other measures) burns, sunburn, and broken bones. Virtually every injury involves blood vessels that are either torn or engorged to the point where they ooze blood or irritant fluids into your tissues. Cold applications shrink those damaged vessels and cut down the amount of leaked-out material your body has to carry away before you get well. So here's the first thing to do with almost every injury:

STEP ONE: Chill sprains, strains, muscle pulls, bruises, burns, and sunburns to get prompt relief and speed healing. Prompt chilling keeps damage from almost any injury to a minimum. Promptness is more important than degree or uniformity: better to use a towel wet at the drinking fountain *NOW* than to wait until you get home to use an ice bag. Use the ice bag too, of course, but don't pass up less efficient but more available methods for even a few minutes in the meanwhile.

When chilling bruises, sprains, and strains, you may need to control the intensity of cold. These injuries do not occasion any increase in blood flow through the part, so over-cooling can cause discomfort or even (in extreme instances) frostbite. Do not pack the injured part directly in chipped ice or its equivalent: put ice in a plastic bag and interpose two or three empty plastic bags for insulation or interpose several moist towels. Or use water out of a cooler, a chemical cold pack, or (last choice) water as cold as you can get it out of the tap.

Burns (including sunburn) instantly draw copious extra blood flow through the injured tissues. The extra circulation reheats the injured tissue faster than even direct ice applications can cool it. You can put crushed ice right on a burn or sunburn. Use towels to keep from freezing the hand with which you are holding the ice in place instead of putting them between the ice and the burned tissue.

How often should you chill an injured part, and for how long should you continue periodic chilling? With burns, you have a built-in index: chill every time the pain (which generally vanishes completely with thorough chilling) comes back. Keep chilling at intervals until no substantial pain recurs. Treat every burn as if it could be a bad one: not even a doctor can tell in the first few minutes which burns will blister, so it's better to be safe than sorry.

Sunburn (if you've ignored my advice about keeping out of those wrinkle-causing rays enough to get one) may involve enough of your body surface that you do better to chill one area at a time. Just rotate one or two plastic bags full of crushed ice from one area to another to keep pain at bay, with a moist towel or two between them and your skin if direct contact with such a large area makes you feel chilled.

Years ago I used to take my five children camping in some rather isolated areas. On one such trip my younger daughter went fishing in an open boat wearing only a bathing suit and came back bright red and miserable. I had only enough ice in the cooler to chill one shoulder and one side of her back, and that for only a few minutes. Even with that sparing application, the chilled side never got beyond mildly uncomfortable pink, while the untreated side actually blistered and took ten days to heal. That thoroughly convinced *me* of the benefit of prompt chilling for sunburn.

There isn't a simple test like pain control that tells you how often and for how long to chill a bruise, sprain, or strain. Chilling doesn't give as much instant pain relief for these conditions as it does for burns, but it's even more important for speeding healing and preventing possible residual lifelong miseries. Almost any injury deserves at least 10 minutes of prompt chilling, and another 10 minutes three times in the next 24 hours. Larger parts need to be chilled longer—a sprained ankle for 15 minutes, a knee or back for perhaps 20. Severe injuries need chilling at least four times a day for at least 48 hours—longer if swelling continues to increase. Chill sprains or strains intermittently for at least 48 hours if you are taking any blood-thinning medications (which interfere with your body's ways of sealing off leaks of fluid into tissue as well as its ways of controlling actual bleeding), including aspirin as recommended in Chapter 1.

There's another side to the need for chilling: it also means *no hot applications, showers, or baths.* As we'll see later in this section, heat helps your body to carry away leaked-out fluid from injured tissues when healing reaches that stage. But it does more harm than good as long as vessels are leaking or oozing irritant fluids into your tissues. If you must shower during the first day or two after an injury, keep the water as cool as you can tolerate and tie an ice bag over the injured area. Don't use heating pads or hot compresses for at least two days after swelling stabilizes.

During a tennis game, Jack R. suddenly felt something snap in his left calf. The pain started a few seconds later, and became steadily more intense until he could barely hobble off the court. Clearly he had torn a muscle trying to make a sudden start.

On my advice, Jack promptly chilled his lower leg with ice bags and avoided hot showers for two days. He was

*able to walk comfortably in one day and got back to
tennis in a week. At that point he thanked me profusely
and explained that he had suffered a similar injury in
his right leg the year before, had gone home to a hot
shower, and been laid up for two months.*

**STEP TWO: Check for fractures whenever bones are tender
to touch or impact.** One of the most damaging old wive's tales
about injuries states that "If it's broken you can't walk on it."
I can't count on my fingers the patients who have walked
into my office with broken leg or hip bones. Wrist and hand
fractures can be even more subtle: I once found a week-old
wrist fracture (of a type notorious for later causing a stiff joint)
when examining a supposedly healthy applicant for insurance.

In deciding whether you need to see a doctor for X rays,
these techniques may help:

- Check for *bony* tenderness. If you sustain an injury, press
  your fingertip against each portion of the bones at the
  sides of your ankle down to their tips. Tenderness located
  at the tip of the bone rather than *below* that point suggests
  a fracture rather than a sprain or strain. Whenever you
  injure your wrist, run your other fingertip along the
  top of the hand bone to which your thumb attaches to
  its upper end. Press firmly against the wrist bones just
  above this spot and move your wrist up and down
  and from side to side. If you find any tenderness in
  that spot, see a doctor.

- Check for changes in contour other than simple swelling
  at the site of injury. Compare the injured extremity with
  its mate, especially with regard to bony knobs and prominences. Any difference between the two sides calls for
  a doctor's evaluation.

- Any pain in the middle of your back, in your neck or
  in either hip after a fall calls for getting someone to
  phone your doctor *before you attempt to get up.*

- After any fall that might have injured a hip, lie flat on your back, stretch both legs out straight, and get someone to check whether your legs are the same length. Hip fractures often jam one portion of bone into another, allowing you to walk and move the part with relatively little pain. The injured bone will later absorb, causing crippling after-effects. Change in leg length is much more reliable than tenderness or ability to walk in deciding the urgency of care. This is especially true if you have any sign of osteoporosis (see Chapter 3).

- As a final check, if no other evidence points toward fracture, check for *transmitted impact or compression tenderness.* If you hold your fingers out straight and tap on the ends of them, impact transmitted along the shafts of the bones will usually cause pain at the site of any fracture of a finger or corresponding hand bone. Making a fist and tapping its end transmits impulses along the axis of the hand bones and may cause pain at the site of a hand or wrist fracture. Thumping on the bottom of the heel usually causes pain in any fracture from above the ankle to the hip. Pressing firmly straight back on the breastbone will cause pain at the site of a fracture anywhere along the course of the upper ribs.

STEP THREE: Speed healing with circulation-aiding measures.
Even prompt chilling doesn't keep some blood and other fluids from seeping into injured tissue. Any protein-filled fluid that remains for more than three weeks is gradually replaced by threads of scar tissue. These tiny strands remain for the rest of your life. They rob your tissues of normal elasticity and sometimes cause aching pain with weather change.

As the years go by, your injuries heal poorly, mainly because sluggish circulation carries away more slowly blood and fluids that have seeped into your tissues. You can aid that circulation in several ways.

- Smooth compression with an elastic bandage cuts congestion in veins and capillaries. Wrap an injured leg with a 4-inch elastic bandage, beginning with two or more turns around the foot at the base of the toes, then taking figure eight turns around the ankle and spiraling up the leg. Bandage an injured knee partly bent with figure eight turns overlapping at the back of the joint. You may need a 6-inch elastic bandage to compress an injured thigh. Start with an anchor turn or two just above the knee and spiral up. Wrap an injured hand or wrist with a 3-inch elastic bandage, starting with figure eight turns around the hand and wrist, then spiraling up the arm.

- Unbandage and elevate the injured part at night. You want blood to run downhill from the injured part to your heart. Put two pillows under your lower leg so that it is raised up but parallel with the floor. That helps gravity to speed flow while relaxing tissues at the back of your knee that pinch key veins when your leg is straight. Elevate an injured arm or hand by putting one pillow across your chest and laying your arm on it.

- Splint any injury near a small joint that movement would disturb. This includes cuts, scrapes, and bruises near any joint. A playing card curled lengthwise around a finger makes a good splint. A curled magazine works for a wrist or elbow. In both instances, bending the material around the body part makes it rigid. Pad the inside if necessary and hold it in place with an elastic or gauze bandage. Home splints for larger joints like ankles and knees are generally good enough only to prevent further injury while you get to a doctor. A pillow with several stiff slats, broomsticks, or the like held along its outer surface with circular bandaging works well.

- Get a helper to massage the parts of the extremity into which vessels from the injury drain. The arm or leg should be elevated and powdered with talc. Your helper should stroke the leg or arm rhythmically toward the heart, starting just above the tender area and transporting blood and lymph out of congested vessels. Two or three minutes of massage twice a day speeds healing, even though the tender area is completely avoided.

PRIME STRETCHER 2

*Avoid loss of capacity during
injury-enforced idleness with special exercises.*

Anyone who has injured a knee needs to build up the strength
of the muscles at the front of his or her thigh. Extra tone in
these muscles braces the knee well enough to keep it stable
even if any one of its ligaments is torn or stretched. When I
took care of football players at the University of Minnesota,
anyone who had a knee injury had to build up his thigh muscles
until he could lift his leg with a 100-pound weight on his
ankle before going back into action.

The team's main trainer, who was known as "Snapper"
Stein, suggested that injured players could be brought back
into action faster if they exercised the *uninjured* thigh. To prove
his point, he got ten healthy players to participate in an ex-
periment. After tests showed that they could lift an average
of 36 pounds at the start of the program, he had them exercise
one leg only. When they could lift 100 pounds with *that* leg,
he tested the *unexercised* one and found that they could lift an
average of over 90 pounds with it!

By starting to exercise the uninjured knee as soon as a
player got hurt, we substantially cut the lost playing time for
these athletes. Using a variation of the same technique, I've
cut the disability time for hundreds of patients since. *Exercising
the uninjured opposite extremity can actually build up the strength
of the injured one* instead of letting it shrink away and weaken.
Such exercise also helps keep muscles in the injured extremity
from shrinking, so casts don't need to be changed as often.
Whether the injured part can't be exercised because it's in a
cast or because of tenderness, you can use this technique to
keep its muscles in shape.

**STEP ONE: Maintain muscle tone in an injured part by
exercising its mate.** For leg injuries, do these three exercises
at least three times a day:

1. Strengthen the muscles at the front of your thigh. *This is the crucial exercise for preserving muscle tone when you have a leg injury. Even if a clumsy cast or other problem makes the other exercises impractical, be sure to do this one.*

   • Sit with your leg out straight in front of you, resting on the floor. Set the muscles at the front of your thigh *hard*, pulling the kneecap up toward your hip, for 5 seconds.

   • Keeping the muscles firm, slowly raise your heel about 4 inches off the floor. Hold the leg in this position for 5 seconds.

   • Let the heel down slowly, keeping the thigh muscles set hard. Maintain the tension in the muscles for another 5 seconds.

   • Rest for 5 seconds.

   • Repeat the cycle ten times.

2. Strengthen the muscles at the back of your thigh.

   • Turn to sit backward on the chair, straddling its back. Place your heel against the bottom end of the chair's leg. Draw your heel back against the chair leg as hard as you can. Continue the firm contraction for a slow count of ten.

   • Relax for 5 seconds, then repeat ten times.

3. Strengthen your calf muscles.

   • Stand on one bare foot, resting your hand against the wall to aid balance. Lift your heel about 2 inches off the floor.

   • Bounce rhythmically on the ball of your foot, neither so high that you leave the ground nor so low that your heel touches, for 30 seconds.

   • Rest 10 seconds, then repeat five times.

If you injure a shoulder, arm, or hand, these exercises with the uninjured extremity help to maintain muscle tone in the injured one:

1. Exercise your hand muscles.
   - Squeeze a tennis ball hard for 10 seconds.
   - Relax for 5 seconds.
   - Repeat ten times.
   - Holding your fingers out straight, press the tops of their tips against the bottom of a table for 10 seconds.
   - Rest for 5 seconds.
   - Repeat ten times.

2. Exercise your biceps.
   - Place your hand under a heavy table of desk. Pull up as hard as you can for 5 seconds.
   - Rest for 5 seconds.
   - Repeat ten times.

3. Exercise your triceps.
   - Place the side of your fist on the top of a table or desk. Press down firmly for 5 seconds.
   - Rest for 5 seconds.
   - Repeat ten times.

Let me tell you about just one case in which exercises of the uninjured limb clearly made a big difference.

At age fifty-three, Lil G. went skiing with her sister at a Utah resort. Her sister went down the advanced ski slope one morning and reported that the snow was perfect and the run magnificent. Lil started down the same slope at about 3 P.M., only to find that the shifted position of the sun had turned several patches into glare ice. Result: a nasty spiral fracture of her shin bone and 12 weeks in a full-leg cast.

Lil's orthopedist expected to have to change her cast at least once and maybe twice as muscle atrophy made it loose. Instead, Lil kept the muscles in her injured leg from changing contour by exercising the good leg, and never needed to have her cast changed. As soon as the cast came off, Lil used measures we'll discuss shortly to loosen up the immobility-stiffened joints. Inside a few weeks, she had resumed her normal active schedule—not skiing, because all the snow had melted, but tennis, golf, gardening, and the rest.

Lil had only a fraction of the disability her orthopedist expected, considering the severity of her fracture. And she never had any of the weather-change rheumatism that would have been expected. While there's no way to be sure of what her course would have been without the exercises, all of us—the orthopedist, Lil and I—agreed that she couldn't have done better, and that the exercises played a big part.

STEP TWO: Maintain mobility of all unconfined body parts while being treated for injury. Unfortunately, the effects of an injury on your body aren't confined to the injured part itself. If your leg is in a cast, many of your activities change. Diminished activity may lead to stiffness in completely uninjured joints. To keep down the time necessary to get back to full activity, you need to pay at least some attention to your body's general well-being and condition.

At least three times a day, you should try to carry every joint in your body through its full range of motion. Be sure your body and muscles are completely warm when you carry out this procedure: stretching cold muscles does more harm than good. Don't use one hand or arm to force joints in the other hand or arm farther than they will move with their own muscles.

STEP THREE: Continue to exercise the uninjured leg or arm as long as discomfort limits exercise of the injured one. After your cast is off, you will probably find that discomfort will limit the amount of exercise you can do with the injured part. Continue to exercise the uninjured mate until you can resume absolutely unimpaired activity.

PRIME STRETCHER 3

*Heal wounds faster through nutritional
support.*

**STEP ONE: While healing any injury, including bruises and
cuts (even those done in the course of surgery), take extra
vitamin C and zinc.** Vitamin C plays a big part in healing
connective tissue, and zinc definitely speeds healing of body
surface tissue. While any well-rounded diet includes some of
both substances, wound healing requires higher than normal
levels of both.

A full glass of orange juice contains about 100 milligrams
(mg.) of vitamin C. Grapefruit and tomato juice are somewhat
less rich sources. Exactly the same effect comes from manu-
factured ascorbic acid, so that vitamin capsules containing 100
mg. or more of that product also meet your needs.

Studies show that over 80 percent of Americans have too
little zinc in their diets. Most of the remaining 20 percent get
most of their zinc from nutritional supplements. You will almost
certainly heal wounds more rapidly if you take enough of a
vitamin-mineral product to provide 15 mg. of zinc per day.
(Almost all my patients have found that they can take multiple
vitamin-mineral capsules containing zinc without getting heartburn or indigestion. Those who have tried to take plain zinc
tablets have very often had these complaints. I can't explain
this, but why fight it?)

My patients generally heal cuts, scrapes, blisters (including
fever blisters), and minor burns about one-third faster when
they take zinc than when they don't. Fast healing decreases
your chance of getting a wound infection that might further
prolong healing and increase scar formation. That makes taking
zinc worthwhile whenever you have a wound or injury. It
will not only help you heal faster, but will prevent some scarring
and stiffness that would otherwise contribute to "feeling your
age" for the rest of your life.

STEP TWO: Ask your doctor about vitamin K injections if you have a fracture and have had any signs of osteoporosis. At this writing, studies suggest that vitamin K helps people with osteoporosis to retain the calcium they need for healing osteoporotic bones. This becomes an issue whenever you have a fracture or have had any operation involving your bones. Since the acid in your stomach destroys most swallowed K, you will need your doctor's help to take it, so you might as well ask him whether further studies have borne out the initial promise of this treatment.

STEP THREE: Heal fractures faster by providing extra calcium. While healing bones, your body needs about as much extra calcium as you could absorb from five full glasses of milk a day. Be sure that you provide this much, from natural foods, from calcium lactate tablets, or from Tums® (see Chapter 3).

PRIME STRETCHER 4

Loosen up previously injured parts with heat and stretching exercises.

If you were a young athlete, physical therapists would barely wait until your injury healed to start rehabilitation. They would use fancy machines to warm tissues, stretch forming fibers of internal scar, and strengthen weakened muscles. They would retrain you to make every movement in a well-balanced way instead of favoring the recently injured part.

For most readers of this book, chances are you won't get anywhere nearly that much attention. In fact, you need this attention worse than a younger accident victim, but experts tend to shrug their shoulders and set very low goals for your rehabilitation. Where they would work to restore a young athlete to his pre-injury status, they'll often be content to get an older man or woman barely out of the rocking chair.

Fortunately, you can do for yourself most of what therapists do for athletes. Most of the fancy machines just deliver *heat*. You can do both the stretching and the strengthening exercises by yourself. A friend can help you to tell whether your body mechanics have changed so that you can take corrective action if necessary.

STEP ONE: Fight post-injury stiffness with heat and stretching. I've kept these measures in one package because *you should stretch a muscle only when it is warm*. It always disturbs me to see my tennis playing friends stretch calf and other muscles just after they walk onto the court. You do absolutely no good and can do harm by stretching a cold muscle. Warm up for 5 minutes or so *first*; then stretch your muscles. If you've had an injury and want to combine rehabilitation with preventing further problems, don't wait until you're ready to exercise. Wait only until the injury has fully healed, so that you can move it without pain and have no local tenderness, before using this method. Also be sure that injury to blood vessels (or preexisting arteriosclerosis) hasn't made heat unsafe by impairing circulation. When these conditions are met, take time every day for a week or more to get the muscle superwarm with heat applications; then stretch it thoroughly.

1. Use a whirlpool bath, hot soak, hot pack, or hot shower through a towel (wrapped around the injured part) to warm thoroughly any muscles and joints that remain stiff after an injury. Water should be between lukewarm and hot—it needn't be as hot as you can stand it. If you add hot water to a soak or compress, always test the temperature with a part that hasn't become used to the heat to be sure you don't burn yourself. The time required to warm the part thoroughly depends on its bulk: a forearm warms in 5 minutes, while a thigh takes about 10. Remember that the muscles controlling movement generally are located nearer to your body than the affected part: you need to warm the forearm before stretching muscles that move your fingers, your whole thigh for stiffness after a knee injury, the muscles of the nearby trunk for stiffness of the shoulder or hip.

2. Carry each injured part through every possible movement five times with its own musculature. For simple hinge joints like your elbow or knee, just flexing and extending the joint suffices. For more complex joints, various types of rotation and other movement may be necessary.

3. For any residual stiffness or restricted movement *except in your elbows or in joints whose further movement is blocked by distorted bone* (use only active exercise—with its own muscles—for an elbow or partially bone-blocked joint), try to extend the range of each possible movement further.

   • Use your other hand to flex or extend fingers, flex, extend, or turn an injured wrist slightly beyond its present limit for 1 or 2 seconds. Relax the pressure and repeat five times.

   • For a stiff shoulder, stand with your chest pressed against a wall. Crawl your fingers up the wall as far as possible, then back down level with your ear. Repeat ten times. Back away from the wall with your upper arm straight out at your side, your elbow bent at a 90° angle, and your forearm extending upward. With your other hand, push your wrist back as far as possible for 5 seconds. Release the pressure for 5 seconds. Repeat five times. Place the back of your hand on the back of your hip. Place the back of your elbow against the wall. Twist your body toward the injured side so that the wall presses firmly against the back of your elbow for 5 seconds. Release the pressure for five seconds. Repeat five times.

   • For a stiff ankle or tight or painful calf muscles, stand with the ball of the injured foot near the edge of a step, with the heel over the step's edge. Put your entire weight on that foot, letting the ankle muscles relax so that the ankle bends sharply and the heel drops below the level of the step. Repeat five times.

- To loosen up the knee area, kneel on that leg at the edge of your bed with the top of that foot flat on the bed's surface close to its near edge. Keep your weight mainly on your other foot, which rests on the floor. Gradually bend the uninjured knee, leaning slightly back, so that your body weight bends your bad knee slightly beyond its prior range. Increase the pressure until it becomes somewhat uncomfortable, then maintain it for 5 seconds. Straighten up for a few moments, then repeat five times.

- Stiffness in an injured hip usually affects rotation more than front-to-back movement. Sit on the edge of a straight chair. With your knee bent at a right angle, put that foot opposite your other hip and turn your lower leg so that the outer edge of your foot is against the floor. Press on the inner surface of your knee with both hands for 10 seconds. Move your foot outward and turn your lower leg so that your foot's inner edge is against the floor. Press on the outer side of your knee with both hands for 10 seconds. Repeat the whole cycle five times.

STEP TWO: Strengthen flabby muscles with isometric exercises. You do isometric exercises without moving any part of your body, by pressing against an immovable object or another body part. This has several advantages for rebuilding strength after an injury.

- Isometric exercises involve no joint movement, so you can start rebuilding strength while discomfort still limits such movement.

- Since no special equipment is required, you can do these exercises any time and any place.

- The fact that they can be done without body movement often lets you exercise while talking on the phone, reading a book, or carrying on a conversation. This lets you do these exercises much more often than varieties that totally interrupt all other activities.

All the exercises I've suggested that you do with the injured part's mate in Prime Stretcher 2's Step One work equally well for the injured part itself, once it has healed enough to make them comfortable. *Strengthening and maintaining the strength of the muscles at the front of your thigh after a knee injury is particularly important.* You can greatly decrease chance of reinjuring your knee by getting in the habit of setting your thigh muscles hard, relaxing and then resetting them every time you get a chance. This not only cuts your chance of reinjury of that knee but also makes you less likely to injure the other one (which otherwise happens quite often).

STEP THREE: Check our own body mechanics. Any injury involving weight-bearing joints (including your back) tends to change your posture and gait. Sometimes these changes persist after the injury has healed, either because you've formed new habits or because of residual tenderness or stiffness. These changes place new strains on your system, often causing discomforts far removed from the site of the original injury. An injured ankle can change your gait so that you get backaches, for instance. Changed body balance can even cause pressure on nerve roots in your neck resulting in pain in the back of your head or in your shoulder and arm.

If you can get someone to help you make certain observations, you may identify such undesirable changes in body mechanics.

1. Bare your back and get your helper to make a mark with a water-soluble felt-tipped pen over the tip of each under-the-skin knob in your spinal column. While you are standing straight, he or she should check to see if these marks form a perfectly straight vertical line. If any S curve or slant is present, check leg length and use wedges to correct any imbalance as described on page 257.

2. Check, preferably by comparing present posture with that in old snapshots, to see if the curves in your spine when viewed from the side have changed. Exaggeration of these curves often changes the position

of your neck in such a way that pinched nerves cause headache or shoulder-arm pain. The posture correction exercises described in Chapter 19 on back troubles may help.

3. If these problems or altered gait, clumsy movement, and so on call for substantial retraining, enlist the aid of a physical therapist.

CHAPTER
22
How to Adjust Medications and Habits to Changing Sensitivities

As the years go by, your body reacts differently to many things. These include

- Alcohol
- Stimulants, including caffeine and its cousins (in tea, cocoa, etc.)
- Medications, both prescription and nonprescription
- Foods
- Vapors, chemicals, and environmental factors
- Internal irritants, like those produced in your tissue by muscle contraction

Unless you recognize and deal with these increased sensitivities, they can make you cantankerous and crabby—qualities one ordinarily associates with age.

PRIME STRETCHER 1

Adjust alcohol use to changed tolerance.

If you drink, you will find as the years go by that the effects of alcohol on your system gradually change. Most such modification stems from changes in circulation and sugar metabolism. Reduced capacity, tendency to get sleepy instead of extra convivial, impaired potency, morning fuzziness, and more intense hangovers all fall into this group.

STEP ONE: Restore capacity with fructose. The only fuel your brain cells ordinarily use is glucose. This "simple sugar" forms from the compound sugars, starches, and proteins you eat and arrives via your circulation. Alcohol exerts its effects by interfering with your brain cells' use of this fuel.

Brain cells can also use fructose, which is a sugar found in certain fruits and in honey. Alcohol doesn't interfere with this process. So you can minimize or cancel the action of alcohol on brain cells with fructose. You can find a pure form of this sugar in your grocery store, or you can use honey (which contains half glucose and half fructose), dried figs, and dates.

You can get fructose into your system by using it in your foods and beverages or replacing ordinary sugars in your recipes. Fructose is a little over twice as sweet as ordinary sugar, so you need to make your cereal, tea, coffee, or desserts very sweet to work substantial amounts into your diet in this way. You can mix fructose into grapefruit juice, lemonade, or limeade.

Your body doesn't store fructose, but if you consume it just before or during a drinking occasion it will generally restore your capacity for alcohol to what it was some years ago. If you overindulge, 2 or 3 ounces will restore coordination in 1 hour and normal blood levels in less than 2 hours.[1] It will also help to minimize hangover.

STEP TWO: Assuage some of the effects of alcohol with vitamin B. As discussed in regard to impotence above, high doses of vitamin B give your system alternate ways of burning sugar. This may help if alcohol impairs potency (although it doesn't usually do much unless you also stop drinking).

---

[1] Without fructose, your body burns about 3/4 ounce of alcohol an hour, and coordination returns proportionately to blood level. This means that an intoxicated person may need as much as eight hours to become fully capable.

Scientific studies have shown that most liver damage linked with alcohol use comes from lack of vitamins. If you replace too much of your body's fuel with beer, wine, or booze, you don't eat enough vitamin-containing food. A well-balanced vitamin-mineral supplement certainly becomes worthwhile.

Vitamin B_1 (thiamine) has been the standard remedy for the neuritis that stems from long-term alcohol use. Ten milligrams a day should ward off this difficulty.

STEP THREE: Avoid morning-after fuzziness by improving fluid balance. To break down one molecule of alcohol, your body consumes eight molecules of water. Unless you replace that loss, the volume of blood circulating through your system decreases. As we discussed in conjunction with air travel, age cuts your body's capacity to adjust to changed blood volume. When you are young, your arteries can change caliber threefold from contracted to dilated, allowing vast adjustment to changed fluid content. When you are older, arteries lose part or almost all of this capacity for changed caliber. Alcohol-caused dehydration lowers your blood volume and diminishes circulation through your brain. Morning-after fuzziness results, often impelling you toward "a hair off the dog that bit you" (which puts you one step farther along the trail toward alcoholism).

You can prevent this effect by supplying your system with plenty of water. The trick is to drink water at frequent intervals throughout the time when your system is burning the alcohol. Unfortunately, just drinking an extra glass at bedtime doesn't do the whole job. Your kidneys clear unused extra fluid through to your bladder within an hour or so, while breakdown of alcohol continues for several more hours. Your system can't recover water from your bladder, so you need a further supply in the middle of the night. Unless you've found that drinking a glass or more of water makes you get up (so that you can drink more) in a couple of hours, you should set a clock or timer and drink another glass or more two hours later if you've had a heavy drinking session.

PRIME STRETCHER 2

Cut down stimulants to control tremors,
anxiety, digestive troubles, and dehydration.

Although Chapter 15 already discussed stimulants with regard to sleep, four other actions of stimulants deserve attention.

STEP ONE: Eliminate stimulants if your head or hands shake. Caffeine and its cousins may aggravate many types of tremor, especially the annoying head and hand tremors sometimes associated with aging. If you suffer from these conditions, it's certainly worth a try to eliminate all stimulants for a few days to see if your tremor gets better.

STEP TWO: Try eliminating stimulants if you feel uptight or nervous. When you have anxiety for any reason, your system makes adrenalin, which tenses you up. Stimulants add to that effect and heighten all its effects—increased pulse and blood pressure, pallor, muscle tension or tremor, and feeling of nervousness.

Why give your system two kicks in the same spot? If you feel anxious, avoid caffeine and its cousins completely.

STEP THREE: Try eliminating stimulants if you have constipation or indigestion. Caffeine and its cousins often cause problems with your digestive system over the years. The amount of stimulant required for this effect is much less than that which affects your nerves, but the time interval is different. What counts to nervousness and lack of sleep is the amount of stimulant you have had in the past 12 hours. What counts to your digestion or bowel function is the amount you have had in the past 3 weeks!

Even two or three cups of coffee or its equivalent per day can cause indigestion or spastic constipation. Caffeine has such varied effects on different people's digestive systems that it's hard to predict what symptoms will develop. If you have heartburn, excess gas, gas cramps, or constipation, try eliminating caffeine and its cousins for a few weeks to see whether you get relief. If symptoms continue, remember that persistent indigestion or change in bowel habit deserve medical attention because of the possibility of a curable tumor. Don't keep trying different home methods without having enough studies to prove no serious disease is present.

STEP FOUR: Eliminate stimulants when your body needs to retain water. We've already discussed how air travel and alcoholic excess deplete your body's blood volume by depriving your system of much needed water. In either instance, caffeine and its cousins do more harm by their fluid-removing action on your kidneys than they do good with their water content.

The other common situation in which stimulant beverages do less good than blander ones is when exercise or plain hot weather has caused you to perspire heavily. If you find that you just don't feel mentally sharp and physically well when you've been sweating, you may have been suffering from internal dehydration. Try rebuilding or maintaining your body's fluids with frequent sips of water, lemonade, or caffeine-free soft drinks, avoiding iced tea, cola drinks, Mountain Dew® or other drinks containing caffeine and its cousins.

PRIME STRETCHER 3

Take smaller doses of various medications as the years go by.

Several body changes related to age make it wise for you to change the dose of either prescription or nonprescription medications you take.

STEP ONE: If you take any medications regularly, check occasionally to see whether you should change dosage. Your body's means of clearing medications out of your system often changes with age. The result may be symptoms of overdosage from an amount you have been taking harmlessly for years. This is especially true of seizure-control medications, sedatives, and blood pressure pills.

Phil S. decided to stop playing tennis at age fifty-two because he was playing too poorly to have a good game with his usual competitors. He found himself sleeping ten hours at night and still feeling tired much of the time, which he blamed on lack of exercise. After this had gone on for almost a year, he developed dizzy spells, which finally drove him to visit my office.

Phil had started taking Dilantin® after having two seizures when he was in his twenties. He had taken the same dosage for almost thirty years and couldn't believe that it had anything to do with his complaints. But studies showed his blood level of Dilantin® was three times what it should be: well up in the toxic range. Adjusting the dosage not only cured his dizzy spells but also restored his coordination and energy. These days he's back on the tennis court several times a week, easily keeping up with his old crowd.

Finally, many sedatives and tranquilizers have different effects on you over the years. A product that used to help you sleep or soothe you may later excite or disturb you. That doesn't mean you've developed worse insomnia or become more nervous—it just means that your aging system reacts differently to medications.

STEP TWO: Take steps to overcome cumulative side effects. Even if you are taking the right dose, blood pressure medications often cause preventable side effects. The products most commonly prescribed for mild hypertension work by removing excess sodium out of your system through your kidneys. In the process they also remove potassium (a similar-structure ion).

Whenever I examined people with no physical complaints, I always asked if they were taking sodium-mobilizing (diuretic) blood pressure medications. If so, even if they weren't aware of any side effects from the medicine, I gave them samples of potassium supplement pills or powders and told them to phone for a prescription if they noted increased energy or other improvement in how they felt. Even though most of them protested that nothing was wrong, most of those who took the supplement called in later for a prescription.

If you are taking blood pressure medication, you can find out whether potassium would make you feel more energetic by including the natural potassium-rich foods listed here for a week or so. This method is impractical for long-range correction of a potassium deficiency, but you can follow it long enough to find out whether you need a supplement. Three pills a day or one glass containing flavored potassium powder contains more potassium than the whole day's allotment of potassium-rich foods in the box, so long-range control of your deficiency with supplements is much easier than using potassium-rich foods. Also, since supplements are prescription products, you may recover the cost from Medicare or your insurance.

Potassium-Rich Diet

Drink with each meal and at bedtime one full glass of
  Orange juice,
  Grapefruit juice, or
  Apricot nectar.
Eat at lunch and dinner one full serving of a leafy green vegetable like
  Spinach,
  Kale, or
  Swiss chard.
Eat at or after each meal a full serving of
  Dried apricots,
  Dried figs, or
  Dates.

PRIME STRETCHER 4

Feel much better by identifying and avoiding foods to which you have become allergic.

Every year that goes by gives your system more chances to develop food allergies. If you get diarrhea, perhaps with cramps, nausea, or heartburn but without fever or general malaise, food allergy is almost certainly the cause. But you might not get any complaints that point to your digestive tract at all! Skin rashes, headaches, muscle pains, fatigue, and other vague complaints can come from food allergy.

If you get diarrhea or nausea from some uncommon food like shellfish, you probably can figure out that you are allergic to it. However, three elements of food allergy make it sometimes difficult to root out.

1. *The most common food allergies are also the most common foods, namely,*

- Wheat.

- Milk and milk products. (This differs from the lactase deficiency that makes 20 percent of blacks and 4 percent of whites get indigestion from whole milk, because it makes cheese, yoghurt, and milk used in cooking also trigger complaints.)

- Eggs.

- The bean family, including black-eyed peas, peanuts, coffee, cocoa, chocolate, and soy sauce.

2. *Symptoms may come on suddenly many hours after you eat the offending food.* Blood tests show that only one food allergy victim in five is sensitive to the undigested protein in the offending food. The rest react to one or another breakdown product formed while that food is being digested. Sometimes that particular breakdown product doesn't form until six or eight hours after digestion starts—often after you've already eaten another meal or two.

3. *You may be able to eat small or moderate amounts of the offending food without symptoms, but become abruptly and seriously ill from just a little more.* Your body has more than one way of digesting many foods. Often you digest moderate amounts in one way, but invoke another digestive path when the preferred route can't handle any more. If the breakdown product to which you are sensitive forms only when your body is using the overload digestive pattern, symptoms may occur only rarely even though you eat the offending food often. This is especially hard to recognize with bean allergy. If you have this condition, you can reach the overload point with any combination of chili con carne, peanuts, chocolate, coffee, and so on, which you don't even think of as similar foods.

STEP ONE: If you know you have food allergies, control whatever symptoms you get with enemas or epsom salts and antihistamines, and check for secondary allergies. It seems obvious that if you know shrimp gives you diarrhea, you shouldn't eat shrimp. But sometimes you'll either try to stay within your limit and fail or eat an appetizer or some soup or a casserole without realizing that it contains shrimp. If that happens, the best way to keep symptoms to a minimum is to get rid of the offending substance quickly. I have had one patient who reacted so severely to shrimp that if he took one bite of something, then realized it had shrimp in it, he would induce vomiting, but most people would find that cure worse than their disease. In most cases, the best way to get the offending food out of your system is with epsom salts or an enema. This may seem like carrying coals to Newcastle when you already have (or expect to get) diarrhea, but it usually speeds relief by getting the offending substance out of your system.

Nonprescription antihistamine allergy medicines like Chlortrimeton® and Benadryl®, both available without a prescription, often give prompt relief. If they're the only ones available for immediate use, you can use hay fever remedies like Allerest®. Since these are compounded mainly for hay fever sufferers, they contain blood vessel shrinking ingredients (for nasal congestion) as well as antihistamines, but a moderate amount of these won't hurt you.

Every attack of food allergy dilates vessels in the lining of your gut and lets undigested and partly digested proteins get into your bloodstream. If your body mistakes those foreign elements in your circulation as invaders (they chemically resemble bacteria and viruses), it will form antibodies and create a secondary allergy. (All allergic reactions stem from your body's use of protective mechanisms it perfectly validly uses against bacteria and viruses against innocent compounds.) Whenever you *know* you have one or more food allergies, chances are you have other *unknown* ones. Particularly if these involve foods you eat every day (like wheat, eggs, milk, and the bean family), you won't know how good you can feel until you eliminate *all* the allergens for a while.

STEP TWO: If you have any reason to suspect food allergy, fast for three days. One of the most common reasons for feeling old before your time is allergy to one of the common foods. If you feel tired all the time, suffer aches and pains, have frequent headaches, have indigestion for which ordinary medical treatment fails to give relief, or have any other possible signs of food allergy, eliminating *all* allergenic foods is the only way to tell whether food allergy is at fault. Blood tests and skin tests by an allergist do no good. As I explained, 80 percent of food allergies involve breakdown products that don't form unless you actually digest the food, while tests always use intact, undigested food proteins. Diary data are unreliable because of the delayed onset of symptoms and tolerance of small amounts of offending foods.

Unless you have some disorder like diabetes that makes fasting hazardous, the ideal way of finding out if you have food allergies is to fast for three days. Drink all the water you want, but eat absolutely nothing. Pick a time when someone will be with you and when you won't have to be very active physically—once in a great while, fasting will lead to dizzy spells or weakness, and you may need assistance. Hunger will usually abate after a few hours, and the rest of the fast will be much more comfortable than you might expect. If you have any food allergies, it will be even better than that—you'll feel 20 years younger!

If fasting isn't practical for some reason, you'll get nearly as good results with the diet explained in the next paragraphs. Only if you're one of the rare people who is allergic to rice or lamb will this make any difference.

STEP THREE: Start from a low-allergen diet and add new foods at three-day intervals to identify the offenders. Perhaps because we eat so little of it, very few Americans are presently allergic to lamb. Rice almost never causes allergy. These two foods supply everything you need to keep healthy and comfortable for a few days. That's what you should eat to sustain yourself while you start on your allergen-discovering quest: *nothing* but rice and lamb, no beverage but water, no seasoning except salt. And *no nutritional supplements!* A large percentage of people who have food allergies are also sensitive to the coloring agents and preservatives commonly used in vitamin capsules.

If you're still feeling as good on rice and lamb as you did while fasting, you can be sure you aren't allergic to either of these foods. Add two new foods, perhaps milk products (including cheese and plain yoghurt) and a favorite vegetable (other than beans). If you continue to feel perfectly well, add two new foods every three days, never including more than one of the most common allergens (wheat, milk, eggs, and beans). Eat plenty of the new foods: you want to be sure to exceed any moderate level that you might tolerate even if larger amounts would cause symptoms.

Whenever you feel less well after introducing two new foods, eliminate both until you feel well again. Don't eat any of the possible offenders until you have found enough proved innocent foods to give a well-rounded, varied diet. Keep a list of all possible offenders and continue to add two more foods every three days.

When you have found enough innocuous foods to be able to eat comfortably both at home and at restaurants, go back to your suspect list. Have epsom salts and antihistamines on hand to help keep any symptoms you precipitate mild. Try small, then medium, then large quantities of each possible offender. It is important to confirm each allergy by provoking symptoms at least once. Otherwise you may severely restrict your diet unnecessarily: I have seen patients eliminate one food after another because they thought they were allergic to it (when they actually had one basic unrecognized allergy or none at all) until they actually had too little remaining variety of food for good nutrition.

PRIME STRETCHER 5

Discover and minimize the impact of environmental factors.

While secondhand tobacco smoke and industrial air pollutants have made a lot of headlines lately, simpler environmental factors that you can readily control cause a lot more misery. If you have a stuffy nose, difficult breathing or continual cough, consider the possibility that something in your environment is causing it.

STEP ONE: Identify respiratory symptoms due to allergy by relief through changed environment or through antihistamine treatment. A stuffy nose or cough that improves when you go on vacation or bothers you more at home than at the office often proves to be allergic. In your fifties or sixties, seasonal allergies like hay fever become less common, and nonseasonal plagues like allergy to dust and molds become more frequent. Any such symptoms that disappear or substantially improve when you take antihistamines are almost certain to be allergic. Removal of airborne particles (see Chapter 20) generally helps.

STEP TWO: Check for formaldehyde. Many new homes use particle board in construction, and most inexpensive furniture is made with bonded wood products. The bonding agent gives off a certain amount of formaldehyde for years—not enough that you can smell it, but enough to cause coughing, and shortness of breath or a stuffy nose if you happen to be sensitive to its action. Such sensitivity definitely increases with age. Often the effects last for days after your exposure ends. You can't tell from the onset of your symptoms whether formaldehyde in your home or office is bothering you. You really need to be away from the troublesome material for a week or more to see if your symptoms clear up.

Sometimes increased ventilation will evacuate enough fumes to make you well. More commonly, you need to get away from the source (or get it away from you) at least for one season. The amount of formaldehyde vapor released falls off year by year, especially if the structure gets warm (in summer) with enough ventilation to let the fumes escape, but I have had at least two patients who simply had to move away from the formaldehyde-producing house.

STEP THREE: Cut the effects of drafts with humidification, lower thermostat setting, or nasal moisturization. One characteristic most people associate with age is sensitivity to drafts. As the years go by, your nasal membranes form less mucus. Dryness makes them react more strongly to air currents. That means you tend to sneeze or suffer stuffiness very quickly when air strikes you.

Complaining about the draft or bundling up might make you seem older to your associates. Why not try to attack the nasal dryness that makes you react to drafts instead of the drafts themselves? Three approaches work well.

- Humidification. If you can put enough moisture in the air to keep the relative humidity up near 50 percent, your nasal lining will stay moist enough to make you less sensitive to drafts. This is almost impossible in cold climates, both because it calls for vaporizing a huge amount of water and because the windows will run with condensate. In milder climates, this might do the trick.

- Lowered thermostat setting. Both chilliness and nasal reaction to drafts is less if you cut the room temperature to the high or mid-60s and wear appropriate clothing.

The main reason for this is actually the effect on relative humidity. Cooling air 5 degrees makes the same amount of moisture twice as effective in raising the relative humidity. (My aunts used to keep the thermostat at over 80°F and suffer from the least, tiniest draft. I measured the relative humidity in their home at 10 percent. Cutting the temperature to 70°F with no added moisture brought the relative humidity up to 40 percent and greatly improved their comfort. At first they wore extra sweaters to compensate for the cold, but ultimately they found that the better heat-humidity balance kept them comfortable with about the same clothing they wore at 80°F.)

- Use moisturizing nasal spray. When I wrote my first book, readers had no choice but to mix their own moisturizing spray with the formula in the accompanying box. Now most drugstores have handy sprayer units. I just bought a generic one (Health Mart's saline nasal spray) at a very low cost. That's a good way to find out what nasal moisturization will do for you. If you find that it makes you much more comfortable in dry, heated air, buy a refillable atomizer and follow the recipe here. A whole pint of solution will only cost a few cents that way, and you'll feel much more inclined to use it freely.

Proetz Solution
(Nasal Moisturizing Spray)

1 tablespoonful glycerin, obtained from any drugstore without a prescription

1½ tablespoonfuls rubbing alcohol

1 teaspoonful table salt

1 pint distilled water (if unavailable use tap water, but let it stand in an open vessel for 12 hours to let chlorine evaporate)

PRIME STRETCHER 6

Control leg cramps due to accumulated lactic acid with vein-flushing exercises, bed cradles, and quinine.

One aggravating complaint that occurs more and more commonly in middle age is leg cramps. These usually occur at night, waking you from a sound sleep. They subside after you get up and hobble around on the crippled foot for a minute or two. Then you go back to bed, hoping you won't get another cramp (which unfortunately sometimes occurs).

STEP ONE: Try vein-flushing exercises to counteract long periods of standing still. If leg cramps occur primarily after you have been on your feet a lot during the day, stand still for 2 minutes (so that leg veins will engorge somewhat) and feel the veins in your lower leg. If one or more is as large as a lead pencil, you have enough vein engorgement to consider the veins "varicose" even if you haven't noticed any enlarged surface veins. In this case try using the vein-flushing exercise described in Chapter 2.

STEP TWO: Buy or make a bed cradle. Nocturnal leg cramps often stop if you keep the weight of the covers off your feet. If you want to find out whether this will help you before investing in purchased equipment, you can make a temporary cradle from two pasteboard cartons. Leave two adjacent sides and the bottom of each box intact while cutting away the remainder to make a cover support for each bottom corner of your bed. Put these supports outside your bed's bottom sheet, but inside its top one so that they hold the covers out of contact with your feet. If night cramps become substantially less frequent, buy a bed cradle at a hospital supply store. A bed cradle has a folding metal strap framework, easily transported or stored. It fits under the top covers at the foot of your bed to make a clear space for your feet.

STEP THREE: Take quinine for ten days, which usually gives six months' relief. Don't ask me how a medicine that your body clears out of your system almost immediately can have such lasting effect. I just don't know! But taking one 5-grain quinine tablet a day for ten days (which you can buy without a prescription in most states) virtually always relieves night cramps and usually wards them off for six months or so.

Quinine was used for many years to ward off malaria, so literally millions of people have taken it safely. If you are a premenopausal woman, time your course of quinine to avoid taking it during your menstrual period (since it might cause increased menstrual cramps) and don't take it if you're pregnant. If you're one of the few people who is extra sensitive to its action, it can cause ringing in your ears (in which case cut the dose in half). *Note that you shouldn't take quinine for day cramps.* Leg cramps that come on immediately when you walk a certain distance generally stem from poor arterial circulation (see Chapter 2). Quinine can make arteries contract, aggravating rather than helping this condition. Otherwise, quinine is quite safe in this dosage.

Dick N. had muscle cramps at night three or four times a week. At age fifty-one, Dick ran a successful sign company, that kept him chained to his desk eight hours a day. To keep in shape, he played tennis (indoors or out) several times a week, and he first came to me because he wondered whether the activity caused his cramps. If so, he planned to give up the game even though it was the keystone of both his fitness program and his social life.

"I just can't take those cramps any more," he told me. "They hurt so bad, they wreck my sleep. And my legs stay sore for hours afterward sometimes."

The day after he started on quinine, his cramps stopped. He completed the ten-day course and quit, expecting the cramps to come back right away. Eight months later he had his first recurrent cramp. He immediately took quinine for another ten days and remained cramp free for over six months.

That was twelve years ago. Last summer I played on the court next to Dick. He waved me over and told me he just takes a course of quinine pills every six months now instead of waiting for the cramps to recur and hasn't had one for years.

———————————

CHAPTER
23
How to Cope with Loss

Along with death and taxes, one other thing is certain: life will deal you at least *some* severe blows. You will lose some things that are really important to you.

- A dear friend or relative may die.

- You may lose an important relationship through divorce or estrangement.

- You may lose the prospect of long-continued life (when you have a terminal illness).

- You may lose a specific capacity, like vision, hearing, or use of some body part.

- You may lose a job, position, or resource important to your feeling of worth.

- You may suddenly become aware that you have lost a level of capability or skill important to your feeling of self-esteem.

You may have read about the five stages of adjustment to a death in the family. The process by which you adjust to other types of loss is exactly the same. Whether confronted with divorce, disability, a dear one's death, or some other major blow, you tend first to dull the shock through *denial*. Then you tend to find something or someone you can blame, using *anger* as a defense against this blow of fate. Ultimately, you feel strong enough to assume responsibility yourself, which imposes a burden of guilt and *depression or mourning*. When you emerge from that stage, you start an *analysis of your remaining assets*.[1] As you learn to use these for a fulfilling life, you become comfortable with your new framework and reach *adjustment*—the state that lets you cope best. The time intervals vary widely, with each phase taking only moments on some occasions and literally years in others.

You should never think of the earlier stages of this process as bad. You may be unable to immediately withstand the shock of your loss and need to work through denial or anger before facing it. These reactions aren't *wrong* or even harmful in themselves. They become so only when they last too long—when they freeze your progress toward something better. Since they shield you from responsibility and guilt, they indefinitely postpone the uncomfortable depression-mourning phase. Once you face the fact that the earlier phases are keeping you from making a more satisfactory long-range adjustment and let yourself mourn, the rest of the process tends to follow.

You can (and probably should) use *denial* and *anger* to keep you comfortable. But you shouldn't let them endure. Ultimately, you need to build your own inner strength or find enough external supports to let you endure the emotional discomfort of *depression and mourning*, which will then both let you move along the path to final adjustment and (by its discomfort) impel you along it.

This process lets you cope with losses that would otherwise make life a burden instead of a joy and lets you emerge still able to make the most of your remaining relationships, circumstances, and capacities. Understanding each stage and what you must do to get past it really helps.

---

[1] Other authors on this subject call this phase "negotiation." The implication is that you bargain with yourself to find trade-offs for the loss, which keeps you looking backward. I feel that you do better to direct your thinking entirely at your remaining assets and how to apply them in building a future.

PRIME STRETCHER 1

*Face facts as the first step toward ultimate
adjustment.*

Your reaction to any really disturbing loss generally starts with
denial. "It can't be true," you say to yourself. "There has to
be something I can do to get back what I've lost."

If there really *is* something you can do, by all means put
most of your energies into restoring your seemingly lost relationship, situation, or capacity. I would feel very badly if any
of my readers took the advice in this chapter as an excuse for
giving up a crucial fight, for saying "Why try counseling?"
when sliding toward a divorce or "What's the use going through
an operation" when faced with a tumor.

Still you need to get past denial as soon as possible. Even
if you need a little time to absorb the shock, prolonging that
interval does considerable harm. As long as you're fighting
against the facts or are devoting yourself to futile efforts to
alter them, you suffer constant anxiety and stall the whole
adjustment process. You can't start to learn to live with your
altered situation until you admit to yourself that you can't
remedy it.

**STEP ONE: If possible, prove the loss to yourself with your
own senses to start the process of adjustment.** Even though
you intellectually accept pronouncements from a reliable source
as fact, they often don't penetrate to the core of your being.
I have seen this most commonly in conjunction with the death
of a dear one. The bereaved widow, widower, parent, or child
nods when told the bad news, but looks dazed and uncertain.
The cruel fact of death doesn't come through until he or she
actually sees the remains. Almost every culture's funeral customs
are based on this fact and include viewings, vigils, or other
such ceremonies. That wouldn't be true unless a vast weight
of experience proved that this observance helps the survivors
get on with their own lives. Two of my experiences have some
bearing:

Glenda G.'s husband's airplane crashed into the sea. Weeks later, she remained dazed and distracted. She just "couldn't believe that he was gone."

Paul C. was out of the country when his mother abruptly died. According to her wishes, she was cremated. Paul remained terribly upset for weeks, saying repeatedly: "There isn't even a grave I can go to."

As unpleasant and stressful as our funeral customs seem, they do bring other concerned people to your side for mutual support while (aided by your own senses) you get past the stage of denial and begin to adjust.

STEP TWO: Sort out and eliminate false hope. One of our society's most harmful old wives' tales is that the best way to help someone through a crisis is to "keep hope alive." This might be justified when there is real hope (especially when it's necessary to remedial action). When it is false hope—when there is no real chance of getting back the lost relationship, circumstance, or capacity—all it does is impose that most unpleasant of emotions, anxiety, and keep progress toward adjustment at zero.

At age twenty-four, Dave T. lost his vision in a hunting accident. When he tells the story, he quotes from the Emergency Room physician's notes, which make it clear that he would never see again. But that's not what anyone told him at the time.

For more than three months, Dave's doctors conspired with his own subconscious to sustain the false idea that he might regain his vision. A blind person often perceives the world as swirling gray instead of black. When Dave talked about that sensation, doctors called it "light perception" even though they knew better. When doctors held up one or three or five fingers in front of him, Dave sometimes could talk himself into considering shadows in the swirling vacuum as vision and naming a number. If he guessed right, everyone made much of it, as if it meant that he was getting back his sight.

Dave is a sweet-tempered person—an accomplished marriage counselor with almost total self-control. But anger and bitterness still creep into his tone when he talks about those days. The constant anxiety—would he ever see again or not? All that time in totally futile straining toward the unreachable goal of restored vision! The overwhelming waste of devoting himself constantly to a battle that everyone else knew from the start he couldn't win!

After almost four months, a rehabilitation technician, not a doctor, finally laid it on the line. He told Dave bluntly that his eyes were useless, and he might as well devote his energies to learning to live without them. With his help Dave did a great job of it and lives a full and useful life, which includes fervent espousal of reality therapy. People can adjust to almost anything, he says, including loss of most future life to a mortal illness. One percent hope is 99 percent anxiety, he maintains, and anxiety is the world's most miserable emotion. False hope leaves you devoted totally to futile efforts to regain your loss, leaving absolute zero for getting on with your life.

Dave convinced me of these points, but it was two years before I got the courage to give his ideas the ultimate test.

Edith R. came to my office for a "checkup," admitting to no complaints or symptoms. After X rays and other studies had shown that Edith had lung cancer, she admitted that she had had a cough for months and coughed up blood before making the appointment. But the idea that she might have cancer frightened her so badly that she wouldn't admit it even to herself.[2]

---

[2] This is another way denial does harm. It reminded me of another patient who endured postmenopausal bleeding for seven years before seeking help, saying: "I know it can't be cancer or I'd already be dead."

All through the losing battle with her disease, Edith suffered almost unbearable tension. She was so afraid! Her hands shook, her skin paled, her eyes darted constantly from thing to thing. When it finally became clear that she would die of her disease, I couldn't believe that she would bear up under the news. But I remembered how strongly Dave felt that the anxiety of falsely hopeful doubt is harder to bear than almost any reality. So I told Edith the grim news.

The next time I saw her, her tremors had disappeared. She hadn't needed a single sleeping pill or tranquilizer. She had made up a list of people she wanted to see and things she wanted to do and started to carry out her plan. She made better and more comfortable use of the time which remained to her than she had of the previous many months.

False hope generates both anxiety and denial. Anxiety is miserable, and denial sidetracks the whole process of adjustment. But the idea that any hope (even if totally unjustified by the facts) will *help* instead of *hurt* your ability to sustain a loss is so ingrained in our society that you may have a hard time getting the facts.

First, you may have to drive yourself to ask the vital question. Time after time I have seen patients have trouble with this. During their first visit, they will say that they want to know the truth no matter what it is. But when studies have been completed and the patients realize you know the answer, they almost never ask the question. They subconsciously find the facts too grim to deliberately pursue.

Don't molder in the morass of denial by dodging the issue. If you seem to have lost crucial prospects or capacities, try to get a straight answer and get on with the process of adjustment.

Second, you may need help from a relative in getting the facts. This is particularly true when doctors are involved.[3] Often your doctor will give your closest relative the facts while he's still painting a different picture for you. Then the only way to get the truth is to have that relative ask questions and relay the answers.

STEP THREE: Focus on your loss to rout denial. You can move on toward adjusting to a loss only when you squarely face one key fact: what the event means to *you* and to *your* future. Not just that your spouse has died or permanently left, but that *you* must live without a husband or wife. Not just that your disease is beyond any hope of cure, but that *you* won't live beyond the next few months. That *you* must live on in a sightless world, or without a familiar, status-assuring job, or without your favorite sport.

This might seem like kicking yourself in an already terribly sore spot. But believe me, you can make the most of whatever remains—but only if you totally acknowledge the loss and its effects on *you*!

PRIME STRETCHER 2

Recognize and understand the anger phase so that you don't get trapped in it.

Once you acknowledge your loss, your next reaction is usually some form of anger. Since yielding to anger has usually been criticized throughout our upbringing and training in manners as "lack of self-control," all of us tend to think of it in terms of one euphemism or another—as resentment, indignation, or

---

[3] Doctors want you to keep trying to rectify the situation instead of resigning yourself to it. Also, they can be sued for being wrong. In one famous case, a patient who was told he had six months to live liquidated all his assets and parceled them out over that period to do all the things he had always wanted to do. When he outlived his predicted span and found himself destitute, he successfully sued the doctor whose prediction had proved pessimistic.

annoyance. That makes recognition of what is *really* going on very important.

STEP ONE: Identify any form of anger for what it is so that you can deal with it. Anger following a major loss often takes one of these forms:

- "Why me?" which indicates general and nonspecific resentment. It stalls the process of adjustment, but at least it doesn't have other harmful effects.

- "A merciful God wouldn't do this" is a form of anger I have seen deprive once-profound believers of their faith just when they needed it most.

- "They [a different race, religion, or gender] did it to me" adds to unfortunate prejudices as well as stalling adjustment.

- "I hate X for it" focuses your anger [perhaps unfairly or harmfully][4] and perpetuates it.

All these forms of anger stir harmful and unpleasant emotions. They often interfere with key relationships. Most of all, they direct your thoughts and energies toward unwholesome blame-fixing rather than the constructive channels that will let you ultimately adjust to your loss and get on with your life. No matter by what name you call it, you need to deal with the anger resulting from any major loss before you can move along the beckoning path to adjustment.

STEP TWO: Figure out why and how this loss has made you angry, which almost always helps you to dissipate it. Although the methods for dissipating anger discussed in Chapter 13 may help, the anger phase of response to major loss often needs something more. You need to examine and understand this phenomenon to deal with it and get on with the process of adjustment.

---

[4] As when one parent blames the other for a child's unpredictable accident.

All forms of anger are *preventive war*. They let you *strike out at someone or something* instead of receiving or acknowledging a blow to your self-esteem. This can be an effective mechanism in some forms of personal interplay, but it is worthless in dealing with irretrievable loss. Even if you strike out at the true cause of your loss, you can never restore the lost person, relationship, prospect, capacity, position, or skill. If anger is misdirected, even greater harm can result.

To get on with the process of adjustment, you need to appreciate the futility of anger and focus on your loss and its effect on your future. Fixing blame gets you no place. Focusing on what you have left—the pieces you need to pick up to get on with your life—accomplishes much more.

Four years after his wife died following a collision with a truck, Jerry P. remained convinced that the common practice among long-distance drivers of using "Bennies" or amphetamines to stay awake was at fault. Police investigation hadn't shown the truck driver to have done anything wrong, and there was no evidence that he had used stimulants. Nevertheless, Jerry devoted every minute of his spare time to campaigns against use of such products by truck drivers. He scanned dozens of publications to collect stimulant-condemning materials, wrote and distributed tracts, and pestered his political representatives at every level.

When Jerry started staying away from work to picket the legislature, his employer asked me to intervene. At first Jerry constantly turned the conversation toward his crusade, while I turned it back to the mourning process and his own adjustment to his wife's death. Ultimately, he broke down in tears and confessed that on the fatal day she had left the house in a pique after an argument with him. He felt very guilty at having "driven her to her death." We talked further about that, and Jerry finally worked out for himself the mechanism by which he had been trapped in the anger phase by subconscious fear that the extra burden of guilt[5] plus the inevitable depression from losing his wife would be too much for him. He still continued his crusade (because he had become so involved in it in the meanwhile) but with far less intensity and not to the exclusion of everything else. Ultimately, he became involved in other things and got back to a balanced and rewarding life-style.

PRIME STRETCHER 3

Let yourself mourn so that you can ultimately cope.

Painful as the mourning process can be, it is the only way to get through to a better adjustment to loss. Some things can make it easier to bear.

STEP ONE: Don't let unjustified guilt add to the burden of your mourning. The most difficult losses are those about which you feel guilty. This usually follows one of two successions of events:

Most commonly, a loved one suffers a long and painful illness. Before the end, you find yourself thinking over and over that he or she would be better off dead and ultimately wishing or praying that the ordeal be over. When death finally comes, the fact that it *follows* your wish seems to some level of your mind as if it had been *caused by* that desire—what psychologists call "wish fulfillment."

This mechanism often imposes such a burden of guilt that mourning and depression become very intense. If you understand what is happening (or has happened), you usually get over the death much more readily.

---

[5] Depression is anger turned inward and is greatly increased by even unjustified feelings of guilt.

Less commonly, either you or a loved one has a severe (not necessarily fatal) accident. Such accidents involve many contributing factors—exact timing, precise location, inattentiveness or distraction, and so on. There are hundreds of ways you can feel guilt at having contributed to one or the other of these: by having had an argument, by having delayed the person's departure, by having asked him or her to run an errand, even by having given him or her something pleasant (but distracting) to think about.

If you find yourself accepting a burden of guilt on some such basis, think the matter through. Certainly these things involve neither intent nor predictability. Should they really instill a feeling of guilt?

You will usually conclude that they shouldn't and become more comfortable.

STEP TWO: Get some of your mourning over in advance if possible. Next to a loss about which you feel guilty, the next hardest to bear is one that is very sudden. Sudden deaths or losses of capacity give you no chance to get any of your mourning over with in advance. The total burden of the loss strikes you in an instant, which is very difficult to bear.

Sometimes there is no way of avoiding this type of blow. Quite often, though, you can "see it coming." You can get the facts when a dear one has a mortal illness. You can ask your doctor what to expect (or the worst case scenario) when you have a disorder likely to impose later limitations. You can ease into retirement's loss of job-related stature.

Perhaps you will occasionally suffer an unnecessary upset by crossing bridges before you come to them. More often, you will soften and make manageable a blow that otherwise would be devastating.

STEP THREE: Express grief as a necessary part of coping with loss. Grief needs an outlet. Whether this takes the form of tears, written or spoken words, or artistic expression of some sort, you cope better with any loss if you can let these feelings out. You need not force the process: Just don't hold back when it happens. Don't let old wives' tales like "it isn't manly to cry" restrain you.

Almost everyone accepts the need to mourn as part of adjustment to the death of a loved one. Unfortunately, relatively few people seem to understand this need in conjunction with the other types of loss we're discussing. A friend who would comfort you through your tears after loss of a dear one will often shrug and grimace when you weep for lost use of a body part or of a relationship. Don't let such misinformed response keep you from expressing your grief, though. Open mourning remains the best and quickest way to get on with your life after any loss, no matter what its nature.

A truly sympathetic person can help you greatly with the mourning process. Just having someone around who cares is a help. If that person accepts uncritically your expressions of grief and shows some empathy with your feelings, he or she gives further support. Some people can get similar aid by communing with their God in prayer if they have sufficient depth of faith.

STEP FOUR: Seek medical help with prolonged or severe depression. One of the world's most poorly defined lines falls between self-limited and generally wholesome mourning on the one hand and morbid depression on the other. Your judgment of whether the intensity of mourning suits the extent of loss is often misleading: a loss that one person finds easy to bear can be much more significant to another. Here are a few examples:

- A wife whose childhood had been plagued by penury and financial insecurity became depressed by a financial loss that didn't upset her husband (reared in an affluent family) at all.

- One woman became tearful and depressed after a fertility-destroying hysterectomy, which her best friend (who had greeted this aspect of a similar operation with joy) couldn't understand.

- A mild heart condition that limited only extreme exertion proved very depressing to a man whose iron-man exercise program had been important to his self-esteem, when most men in his age group would have shrugged it off as unimportant to their life-style.

Instead of trying to determine need for antidepressant medications or care on the basis of the apparent aptness of the response, use the following list as a basis. If three or more of these elements is present, it makes sense to treat the situation as morbid depression (which both requires and generally benefits greatly from treatment) rather than self-limited and wholesome mourning:

- Insomnia, especially waking in the early hours and being unable to get back to sleep.
- Weight loss with loss of appetite.
- Constipation.
- Crying, especially when alone.
- Intensified blue feeling in the morning. Morbid depression often makes you feel as if you just can't face the day when you first get up, even if the blues are more tolerable as the day wears on.
- Suicidal thoughts. Vague feelings that life isn't worth living or asking yourself whether you should end it all deserve attention if any of the preceding elements are present. Thoughts involving concrete methods like jumping off a bridge, shooting yourself, or taking poison deserve attention even if none of the other elements are present.

If you or someone important to you seems to have gone beyond normal mourning into morbid depression, doctors can help. This type of depression doesn't come from weakness or inability to cope. It involves an abnormality in the way nerve impulses move through the brain.

When one brain cell stimulates a neighbor, it does so by squirting out a chemical. A different chemical then neutralizes this stimulus carrier so that its action doesn't make the neighbor cell keep firing over and over. At least eight different stimulus chemicals and corresponding neutralizers operate in different parts of the brain. The pair operating in the emotion-governing portions are *dopamine* and *dopaminase*. Depression results when lack of dopaminase permits dopamine to make neighbor emotion-generating cells fire over and over, almost ceaselessly.

You can fight coping difficulties with understanding, with better coping methods, with external support, and perhaps with faith. To fight chemical abnormalities you need therapeutic chemical agents. Don't hesitate to ask your doctor for medication (and to take it) if signs point toward morbid types of depression instead of ordinary mourning. And don't lose patience: the best antidepressant medications take several weeks to take full effect, so stick with any prescribed program until it has time to work.

PRIME STRETCHER 4

Inventory remaining relationships, assets, and capacities as the basis for a new life-style plan.

When you feel yourself pulling out of the mourning phase after a big personal loss, take time to identify everything you have to work with in building a new life-style.

STEP ONE: Consider your remaining relationships and capacities. When you begin to emerge from the depths of mourning or depression, you need to focus on *assets*, not liabilities. Many of the most important aids to a new life-style don't appear on any balance sheet. Your family, your friends, connections, and activities through which you can expect to make new friends, your remaining capacities and skills—you tend to take all these things for granted. Sit down with pencil and paper and list all of them, besides key possessions and positions.

STEP TWO: Define the worst case scenario. This might seem like focusing on the hole instead of the doughnut, but it usually doesn't work that way. In getting past the remaining vestiges of mourning, it's often a big help to know that the worst things can get will still leave you with a reasonable life-style (which it almost always will). That gives you an acceptable base upon which to build—to devise improvements without concern that you just won't be able to cope.

STEP THREE: Set reasonable intermediate goals. It takes time to develop and round out a new life-style after a major loss. You need a way of experiencing success in the meanwhile. Intermediate goals give you something to shoot at *and to achieve* along the way.

What kind of goals?

- Making some specific number of contacts with family members or old friends

- Resuming or developing a certain number (even one) of socializing activities

- Writing up a realistic budget

- Establishing a health maintenance program—exercise, diet, and so on—to fit your new circumstances

- Revamping your quarters, wardrobe, transportation facilities, and so on, if necessary

STEP FOUR: Try to develop something you can anticipate. Whether it's a visit to a favorite relative or a night school course in a subject you've longed to pursue or a trip to your favorite art museum, something to anticipate helps focus your mind on the future instead of the past. Then it's just a matter of broadening that first bridgehead. Once you have anticipations and pleasant expectations, you'll find the image of a future life-style expanding in your consciousness. You'll find yourself more and more comfortable with your prospects. You'll find yourself adjusting more and more, and finally coping fully with your loss.

PRIME STRETCHER 5

*Let coping methods and techniques help you
even when your loss isn't inevitable.*

Most of this section applies most obviously when a loss has
already occurred or is inevitable. When your spouse dies, you
have no alternative but to concentrate on coping with that
loss.

In many other situations, coping technique can help you
even before the loss becomes certain. When you find that you
have a possibly mortal illness, for instance, you need to deal
with the resulting loss of security even while you take action
against the threat to continued life.

When I found that I had a cancer of the prostate, for
instance, I found myself reacting to the worst case scenario.
This wasn't immediate pain-racked death—I knew that even
if curative treatment failed, available measures would offer me
some comfortable and useful years. I mourned—there were times
when I cried for the possible lost years. I wrote to my children
to tell them how proud I was of them and that my life's
rewards (of which the privilege of watching them grow into
upstanding citizens was the greatest) were certainly all anyone
could expect or deserve. My mourning was over and I felt
comfortable with whatever fate might develop long before I
arrived at the operating room.

The worst case scenario didn't develop. Surgery failed,
but radiation cured the disease. But having dealt with the worst
case kept me calm and unafraid through the whole ordeal.

I certainly hope that you will not need to fight such battles
on two fronts—to cope with the prospect of fearsome loss while
still battling a major threat. But if you do, remember that divide
and conquer works. You can cope with one loss while you
combat another threat. Facing facts—getting past denial and
anger, letting grief flow out through open mourning, and thinking
through the life-style you can develop with the assets that
remain—can minimize the impact of one threat or loss and
free your personal resources to deal with another.

Index